RC
523
.S49
1983

Seymour, Claire.

Precipice

DISCARD

PRECIPICE

Learning to Live with Alzheimer's Disease

by

CLAIRE SEYMOUR

VANTAGE PRESS
New York / Washington / Atlanta
Los Angeles / Chicago

Precipice is dedicated to all those who have walked this path with a beloved relative who suffers from mental illness or organic brain disease. I share my experience and the ways in which I found strength in the hope that it may be of help and comfort to those who have to travel the same tragic journey.

"To appoint unto them that mourn in Zion, to give unto them beauty for ashes, the oil of joy for mourning, the garment of praise for the spirit of heaviness; that they might be called trees of righteousness, the planting of the Lord, that he might be glorified." (Isaiah 61:3)

This book is written to the glory of Him who overcame death, who snatched victory from the jaws of defeat, and by so doing has given us the inexpressibly wonderful privilege of victory in the same circumstances—and above all, the promise and the gift of eternal life.

And When I Die

And when I die,
who will mourn;
and when I pass
from here to there,
who will see me go?
I would rather fall
as a spent ash does,
feather
petal
down,
quelled between two hands of wind;
a broken space,
a sway of time,
no footprints
or apology.
I would rather fall
as a star does
without a slip of sound,
a free-fall way
to something else,
leaving behind
a thin trail of light
that wasn't mine
to begin with.

Pat Waalkes
3-25-77

CONTENTS

Foreword

A close friend with whom the author grew up writes:

This is a story of human tragedy, courage, and love—each one in turn being completely influenced by the author's pure and indomitable devotion to her Creator and her husband.

Later, in her search for help, she found comfort in the efforts medical science is making to find a cure (yet unknown) for Alzheimer's Disease, and the valiant and devoted nursing care at the V.A. Hospitals in Roseburg, Oregon and Tacoma, Washington.

It is a story of sheer heroism—the comfort she brings to to Dave, the sacrifices unmentioned, sorrows overcome, and, throughout, a glowing light between them and their Maker which in the end will conquer all and leave their love unscarred.

Because of the desperate need to help others in the same situation, this will be invaluable.

The book is one of the most compassionate and vital of our time.

B.R.K.
October 1981

1. *Warnings*

This story begins in 1974 and runs up to the present. It is true, for during those years I have had to watch my husband go slowly downhill from Alzheimer's Disease—an organic brain syndrome the cause of which is not yet known and for which there is no cure.

In February of that year, Dave was working as an auditor and investigator for the Oregon Real Estate Division, a job which he had held since June of 1971. The Real Estate Division is a part of the Oregon Department of Commerce, and is the agency which enforces the laws governing real-estate transactions and practices.

The work involved being sent out by the week to different parts of the state to audit the accounts of real-estate brokers and check on the general status of their offices so far as ethics are concerned. It was a job he enjoyed; he had always had a flair for figures and a strong sense of ethics so it was a "natural" for him.

That third week in February, he had been working over in eastern Oregon, and had called me to say that he had "a new addition to the family." Since we had no children at home, this meant that he had found a stray dog. It was an English setter which he had seen running by the freeway with a pack of other dogs. He had watched her all week, and told me that he had tried to catch her by throwing her scraps of meat, but with no success as she was so wild and terrified of people. It appeared that she had been dumped out of a car and abandoned. Eventually, the dog control caught her for him, and he brought her home in a half-starved condition—a fearful, cowed slip of a dog with every bone showing through her skin. She was so dirty that he had to take her in for a bath and trim, and left her in the kennel over the weekend so that this could be done. I mention this episode as it was to become common during the next couple of years and seemed to go along with other signs of deterioration I noticed. This overconcern for stray animals was already beginning to affect his work, although I didn't know it then.

Lately, there had been other instances of a certain disconnectedness with events in the here and now. He seemed to be living on a different wavelength and sometimes appeared not to tune in to the world of reality. I felt sure it was an emotional reaction to his father's death in 1973.

It is now the morning after Washington's Birthday, 1974, and Dave is getting ready to leave for work. Suddenly chaos hits. He cannot find his wallet, his glasses, or his keys. We comb the house, pulling out drawers, looking under the bed, in the pillowcases, under sofa cushions, even in his shoes. For a long time, he has had the habit of tucking these things away in odd and different places, then forgetting where he left them. But this morning, I notice something else. While we are searching, he seems to forget what he is doing—what were we looking for? There seems to be a sort of inability to concentrate, to keep his mind on the search.

He has to call Worth Bellamy, his boss, to explain the situation, and Worth, in his usual patient manner, is sympathetic and understanding. I feel so embarrassed for Dave that I am close to tears and anger by the time he leaves, very late, having stopped payment on the lost credit cards in his wallet.

I spend a laborious day at home. It is gray, foggy, and pouring rain. Everything seems to need cleaning. I have never wanted a long-haired dog, and I feel resentment because he didn't ask me first before bringing her home. She sheds her white hairs everywhere, adding to the general frustrations of that day—the kind of day when I never seem to finish or get on top of things. Deep down, I know that I am upset over his lapse. What could

2

be wrong? He has always been forgetful to some extent, but why this? I don't want to believe that there could be something wrong, so I rationalize and write it off, telling myself that it's the kind of thing that could happen to anyone. Perhaps his mind was preoccupied with other things.

Characteristic of this disease is the fact that in between lapses, things return completely to normal, giving even more reason to think that the forgetfulness was not serious in any way. Twice, however, during the next two months, there were other incidents concerning stray dogs. On one occasion, he picked up a white poodle, again in an emaciated, dirty condition. At first, he didn't tell me, but lodged it in a boarding kennel for several days. Then of course, since this was getting expensive, he wanted to bring it home and keep it. Since we already had two dogs, I protested and was met with violent opposition to the extent that "even if it split up our marriage" he would persist in his rescue missions. I insisted that the dog go to the Humane Society for adoption, and took it there myself. They held it for a week, and meanwhile Dave, who was again working in eastern Oregon, called long distance telling them to hold the dog in his name. He had been checking the newspapers for lost dogs answering the poodle's description, and came home one evening with an advertisement that matched identically.

He seemed to have a kind of intuition that this was the right number, and sure enough, when I called, the lady who answered said that the dog belonged to her granddaughters. They had been moving house one weekend, and in all the confusion the dog had wandered away unnoticed. So, in spite of everything, this rescue mission had a happy ending. The faces of the two children when they saw their beloved poodle were ecstatic, and the dog was no less so. They offered us a reward which we did not accept.

His preoccupation with stray dogs and cats seemed to turn into an obsession, and he must have wasted many hours chasing them and neglecting his work. This was beginning to show because there would be many miles on his car and little or no business to show for it. There seemed to be no way I could get through to him—to make him see that his work was more im-

3

portant than stray animals, however pathetic they might be. Sometimes there was a strange and terrifying barrier in his receptiveness to my feelings, like a blank wall that didn't register.

In July of 1974, he was sent down to the coast for a week to do audits in several different towns. He came back very depressed; he said that he had had a terrible week, but wouldn't elaborate beyond that. Much later, Worth told me that when they read the meter on his car after he returned, there were 721 miles on it and he had only completed six audits during that week. On the surface, it looked as though he had been enjoying himself and doing nothing at the state's expense, but this was probably the beginning of getting lost in places which had always been familiar, forgetting what he was supposed to do, and possibly more distraction due to stray animals.

Vinton Green, a good friend who also worked in the Real Estate Division, told me that Dave had been a problem for some time. He could not keep to his daily schedule of office visits, would do them out of sequence or sometimes forget altogether. He also called on the same office twice within a short length of time to do an audit, having completely forgotten that he'd recently been there. Another weakness was that he hated to write violations. Dave was a sensitive, compassionate person, and rather than write a violation, he would point out the offense verbally to the broker and give him a warning. But the violation would not appear on the weekly sheets he had to turn in to his boss, and he was often in trouble in this respect. Apparently, Bill LaVance, boss of the head office in Salem, wanted to fire Dave, but Worth and Vinton stood by him and persuaded Bill to give him another chance. They both felt that his strange actions were not intentional, but something that was beyond his control.

In August, Bill called him in to the office one day, confronted him with his unsatisfactory work record, and warned him that if it continued, he would be fired. That weekend, we went down to the coast for two nights. In spite of the warning from Bill, Dave was more relaxed and at peace than I had seen him for some time. He was kind, gentle, and considerate of me. He seemed relieved to have had this confrontation about his work.

4

Perhaps it had been a relief to get it out in the open—he may have felt guilty knowing that he was doing an inadequate job, yet not being able to express it or define it for himself. He said to me, "I think my days at the Real Estate Division are numbered." I admired the way he accepted this warning, seeming to understand that it was justified without feeling any bitterness. Nevertheless, I felt real sadness for him because the job had been so well suited to him and for the first two years his work had been excellent. I felt really close to him that weekend in a way that was very special.

Thanksgiving of 1974 was spent with Dave's mother in Oakland, California. Charlie, a long-time friend of Dave's, was also staying for the holiday weekend. The day after Thanksgiving, the three of us took off for an afternoon in San Francisco. We took the bus over, and after walking for a while and doing some window shopping, we ended up at the Marines Club for a drink. The mood was relaxed and jovial between the three of us. Dave and Charlie ribbed each other as usual. In character, they are almost totally opposite. Dave is a deeply private person, never pushes himself on anyone, and can be shy and retiring in a social setting. By contrast, Charlie is a complete extrovert with a big ego— warm, generous, and loves the limelight in any situation.

I don't remember what was said, but our happy conversation suddenly ended and a pall seemed to fall on us. Charlie noticed it too and asked what was wrong. I remember a cold, depressed atmosphere surrounding us—and that we were trying unsuccessfully to recapture the happiness that had so mysteriously slipped away. Eventually, Charlie suggested we go to dinner at a well-known seafood restaurant, and Dave reluctantly agreed. All his enthusiasm for our time out together seemed to have vanished. All through dinner he was quiet, moody, and unresponsive. Usually he would enjoy Charlie's company and laugh at his jokes, but this time he seemed to want to fade out of the picture altogether.

After dinner we went into a department store nearby and were browsing in the jewelry department when we suddenly realized that Dave was no longer with us. A search for two or three blocks proved fruitless, so we went back and waited for him out in front, feeling sure he would soon be back, but with no result.

I felt a heavy load descending on me. I had to make the most of Charlie's company while at the same time making excuses for Dave. Fortunately, Charlie knew him well enough to be familiar with some of his moods. But this was truly outrageous, being discourteous to a guest he had invited for the weekend. The evening deteriorated still further as Charlie and I got separated due to a misunderstanding at the bus station, and there followed a lonely, anxious ride home wondering what on earth had happened to a day that had started with so much promise. Dave was home when I arrived. I never knew what he told his mother, but she handled the whole thing with her usual insight and understanding. I often think she must have suspected then that there was something wrong with Dave. She was certainly perceptive enough. Whatever she may have thought, her attitude was a beautiful example of "pouring oil on troubled waters." When I look back on the whole affair, it is quite possible that Dave genuinely got lost and was not able to find us again. Then, feeling insecure and fearful, he may have got a taxi to the bus station and come home from there. If this was true, he could well have been too embarrassed to admit it. Apologies were made to Charlie, and with Grandma's help reconciliation and forgiveness prevailed, and the evening was salvaged somehow.

Following this incident, there was quite a long period when he appeared to be perfectly normal. Always one who was able to put up a good public front, he may, in the earlier stages, have been able to cover up when he felt himself slipping. During the next few months, he mentioned changing his job several times, and did actually fill out an application for a job with the state Motor Vehicle Department, but didn't follow through as the salary was much lower. It was at about this time too, that I first noticed he would come home from work at odd hours—sometimes as early as 3:30 or 4 P.M., when normally his day didn't finish till five—saying he had made all his office calls for that day. Occasionally, he would drop in during the morning, park his state car in the driveway, and say he had to make some phone calls as he was doing audits in the area. Although I never suspected it then, this must have been another sign of forgetfulness in knowing where he was supposed to be, and at what time. So he really came home to recheck his schedule because he'd forgotten it since leaving the office.

At this time also, he started taking the bus to the office, rather than driving his car. It seemed a logical move since the bus ride was convenient and he always had the use of a state car for work. I remember that he seemed much more relaxed when taking the bus in the mornings than when he drove. Never able to confide his feelings easily, he would often come home obviously depressed. I could tell by his expression and general attitude that the day had not gone well, but when questioned about it he would not go into any depth, so I would pass it off thinking that perhaps it was more his mood than the actual happenings of the day that was to blame.

About the second week of April 1975, I had a gruesome nightmare and woke up with a feeling of doom and premonition. In the dream, I had had a call from the agency where I did volunteer counseling to come down at once. Dave was at the front desk creating havoc. Shouting, tearing up papers, and no one could cope with him. Father Abbott, the executive director, had come downstairs and was speaking to Dave, trying to calm him, but to no avail. He turned around and started to run up the stairs to the second floor, still shouting and totally uncontrollable—immune to any approach. Then I arrived on the scene. I pursued Dave up the first flight of stairs, pleading with him, begging him to stop and come home with me. He looked back wild-eyed, as though I were a complete stranger, and went on up the next flight of stairs to the third floor. I followed behind up the narrow, winding staircase, desperately trying to reach him—to get through to him, stop him somehow, any way I could. As he reached the top, he gradually vanished, faded from sight, and I remember a hopeless feeling—that he was slipping from me and that there was nothing I could do about it. There was a ghastly finality about the whole thing, and I awoke convinced it had actually happened.

About an hour later, a close friend, Gwen, called me to ask

if I was all right. During her meditation time that morning she had felt an urgent conviction that something was wrong, and to get in touch at once. I told her about the dream. Gwen had been a good friend for several years, but from that time on our friendship moved to a really deep level, a totally new dimension of closeness. In the years ahead, she was to be the one to whom I turned most often and who was always there in time of need.

By contrast, this April day was superbly beautiful. It was bright, sunny, and clear, with the trees bursting into leaf, azaleas and dogwood in blossom, full of the promise of new life and renewal that always comes at this time of year. Gradually, throughout the day, my nightmare faded and I remember making a conscious effort to drown it in the company of two good friends, and in the sharing of jokes only the three of us would understand.

Just over two weeks later, on April 29, Dave's mother died. At about 2:00 P.M., his sister called with the news. It didn't register at first—just a kind of dazed numbness, and hearing myself saying automatically all the usual kind of things one says to fill the awful void. I remember thinking I must keep busy—I mustn't stop to think or feel, so I went out and gardened, frantically mowing both lawns. The reality of what I had just heard was beginning to dawn slowly, though the tears had not come yet. The thing I dreaded most was telling Dave—how was I ever going to break it to him? If he reacted as emotionally as he had to his father's death, it might break him completely. So often I had had the feeling that I should try and cushion him from the blows of life—I don't know why—but perhaps it was an instinct that in his life there had been so many setbacks that one more might just be overwhelming. And then there was my own grief. She had been so much to me: mother, friend, spiritual guide, inspiration, comfort. I had always dreaded the day when this would happen; now it was here and had to be faced.

Once more I turned to Gwen. When she answered the phone, I spoke nonchalantly, not knowing how to get to the point. Eventually . . . "I called to tell you that Grandma died today." As I spoke the words, tears could no longer be controlled and it was almost impossible to speak without sobbing. Gwen asked if she should come over to be with me, but I said, "No, just pray for us; pray that I'll be given the right words when I tell him." Dave came home later than usual that day and the agony of waiting seemed like an eternity. I managed to blurt out the news and once again broke down. Surprisingly, he didn't seem to be as upset as I had expected, or at least didn't show it. He made plans to fly down to Oakland later that evening. I was to follow the next day, having put our dogs in the kennel and made arrangements for the mail and papers to be stopped. I remember he said: "I would like Charlie to sing at the funeral," but having talked to Ruth, his sister, who had already made most of the arrangements, he didn't pursue it any further.

The following morning, I was getting ready to leave the house and catch a midday plane to Oakland when Worth called. He asked if I had Dave's briefcase handy, as he wanted to go over some of the reports that had been turned in that week. He told me what he was looking for on the yellow sheets—mostly notations of violations in the various offices which Dave had covered. Apparently, many of the reports were incomplete or did not have the right notations entered. He sounded really worried, and kept me on the phone for about fifteen minutes. I then told him I had a plane to catch and thought he would understand as of course he knew about the funeral. However, he asked if I would have time to come in to the office on the way to the airport. By this time, I felt irritated by his persistence; it seemed such an inappropriate time to have to go over these things; surely he must understand my own emotional state at this moment, so I told him that I was sorry, but there wouldn't be time to do that.

Somewhat reluctantly, he gave in, but said to be sure and tell Dave to get in touch immediately when he got back from the funeral. Worth said nothing to me in this conversation about Dave again being in trouble, but I discovered later that Bill had been pestering him about these unsatisfactory records, and had again pressured him to get rid of Dave, which he refused to do. What a loyal friend. Not only did he stand up for Dave, knowing that his work was much below par, but he never burdened me with the unpleasant news and the pressure he was under from

9

Bill. Doubtless, he wanted me to come into the office that day to talk about this problem.

Going down to stay for the last time in my mother-in-law's house which so recently had been full of her presence, was a nightmare. There were reminders and associations everywhere. Dave and I stayed alone in the house that had meant so much to us both.

I dreaded the funeral and lunch party which had been arranged afterwards, but there were consolations in that Ruth and Nolan handled everything beautifully. Nolan kept everyone going with his cheerful, friendly spirit. I never saw him show any grief openly, so I couldn't help but wonder if he ever expressed it privately.

It was a deeply emotional time. Grandma had touched so many lives and had always been such a cohesive force within the family. Both she and George, Dave's dad, had been in-laws that I loved and respected. They were the personification of love and stability; if any problem arose within the family, they were always the first ones there ready to help in any way possible. I knew I could always count on being welcome at this house on Oakmont Avenue—a place where so many happy times had been spent. Times of hospitality, of deep sharing, of fun and laughter. I count it a privilege to have been a part of that family and to have known, for the past eleven years, these two fantastic people.

As I remember, the funeral was on a Friday. Then on Sunday, there was a memorial service given by members of her own church—a group of about twelve or so. It is this service which stands out in my mind. The spring sunshine poured in through the windows and a mockingbird sang in the background as Marion Johns, a lifelong friend, read from Psalm 103:

Bless the Lord, O my soul and forget not all his benefits
Who forgiveth all thine iniquities; who healeth all thy
    diseases;
Who redeemeth thy life from destruction;
Who crowneth thee with loving kindness and tender
    mercies. . . .

This had been one of her favorites, particularly in the few weeks before she died. In fact, she had said in a letter to us a short time before, "Note the five verbs in this psalm, and the promises they contain."

There was a hushed, reverent silence, broken only by the mockingbird's song, as Marion continued to read. He seemed to be trying to join us and add his own eulogy in remembrance of this beloved friend whose life had been lived in service to others.

Dave stayed on an extra couple of days, and I returned home on Monday. On the whole, he held up much better than I did. I remember coming down to breakfast one morning in the sunny, blue and white kitchen where we had had so many happy breakfasts in the past. The overwhelming truth that they were both now gone hit me hard, and Dave urged me to go home. He was very tender and understanding of my tears.

Once home again, I had a feeling that he was not going to stay in his job much longer, although he needed it all the more now to bring fulfillment and interest into his life. While his mother had been alive it had seemed to be her restraining influence that had kept him in the job, but now that anchor was gone.

Late July was hot and oppressive. The last week of that month, Dave was auditing down in Eugene, about 100 miles south of where we lived. While he was gone, I had been painting the kitchen and back porch, and one sultry evening he called from his hotel sounding really low. He wished so much he was home—the hotel was hot and uncomfortable, and for him it had been a disastrous week. He had locked himself out of his car, had lost the keys and an important check. He had apparently told Bill what had happened, and it didn't take much imagination to guess what Bill's reaction had been. About three weeks later, on August 15, Dave resigned from the Real Estate Division. He had been talking about it openly now for quite some days, so it came as no surprise. It was a Sunday afternoon when he called Bill at home and told him of his decision. I knew it was inevitable under the circumstances, and to have stayed on in the job, pretending that he could still handle it when in reality he couldn't, would have been more traumatic for all concerned.

He must have known by now that something was seriously wrong with him, and that he could no longer function responsibly. Naturally, I felt depressed about the loss; it had been the one job during our marriage that he had really enjoyed and taken hold of with enthusiasm. Worth told me that when he first started, he was very easy to teach, and picked up the details of what he had to do almost at once. In fact, he said it was a pleasure to teach someone who was so quick to understand. In addition, he had made two outstanding friends in Worth and Vinton Green. He had held this job for just over four years and if this illness had not intervened, I am sure he would have stayed on for at least several years more and perhaps permanently.

His resignation did not become effective until September 1st, so he decided to take the following week off and go down to Oakland to help Ruth with his mother's affairs, and was to be gone for the rest of that week.

That same Monday, I left to go down to the coast for a few days. I needed to get away for a while to try and sort out my own feelings about what was happening to us. I remember praying in agony for him, because by this time I was well aware that the future was going to be rough. I couldn't define it, but a deep inner premonition now seemed to be fulfilled, as though I had known inwardly for a long time that this was going to happen. I asked for strength for whatever we might have to face; for courage to face a future which for both of us looked bleak and without promise. I asked that he might be guided to the right job; that his life might find true fulfillment in some way. More than ever, I sensed my utter helplessness and dependence upon God in such circumstances. The whole thing was growing to overwhelming proportions—altogether too big for me to handle.

One of the things in our marriage which had been most difficult for me was his apparent inability to stay with a job for any length of time. In the past eleven years he had changed jobs eight times, with many periods in between when he was doing nothing at all. He had always done well in any courses or exams he took, and had no difficulty at all getting his real-estate salesman's license, and then his broker's license two years later. But it was in applying this knowledge in a practical way that the difficulty seemed to lie. He was fearful of going out as a salesman to sell property, and it was true that he didn't have the necessary drive and aggressiveness for sales. So when this job came up in the real-estate division, it seemed the answer that we had searched for for so long. Now this was over too, and I had to face the fact that he might never succeed, at least in the eyes of the world. To live with the failure of someone I loved and all that this implied—this was what I faced. A path I would never have chosen for myself. Something which happens to "other people," not to us. At times like these the unknown future stretches away full of the threats of disaster. Always in marriage, we assume that it will turn out "for better"; the possibility of "for worse" is pushed out of sight into the background. It is the thing we face last, most reluctantly, and almost never realistically until it is thrust upon us.

Dave returned from Oakland the following weekend, having one more week to work until his resignation became effective. He was extremely reluctant even to come back so as to be in his office on Monday, but I managed to talk him into it. Following the Labor Day weekend, we were to leave again to help Ruth finish cleaning up his mother's house, which had now been sold. There was still furniture to be sorted out between the family and arrangements to be made for the moving and sale of various items.

When we arrived, he insisted on staying in his parents' house alone, rather than with Ruth, where I stayed. His loyalty and association to that house must have been stronger than any of us knew. Perhaps this place where he had spent so many years was the last anchor in his life now with both his parents gone and the loss of his job.

While cleaning out the house, Ruth and I noticed that he was restless, disorganized, and not much help at all. He would go through old papers, photos, or souvenirs, put them aside, then pick them up and walk off to another room where he would be distracted by something else and promptly lose track of what he

13

was doing. He wandered in and out aimlessly and had great difficulty making decisions as to which pieces of furniture he wanted to take.

Shortly now, he was to lose this house too, and in fact his whole life seemed to have been a series of losses, starting with his birth, for Dave was an adopted child. He had been found abandoned in a car park when only a few days old with a note pinned to his blanket, "My name is George Frederick Doe. I need a good Christian home." From there he had been taken to the Y.M.C.A. children's home, and a few months later had been adopted by George and Dorothea Seymour, who saved his life from tragedy, gave him the best possible start they could, and showered him with love and a stable home background.

His mother told me that he had been a sickly baby to begin with, doubtless due to the shock of being abandoned; he was hard to feed and had wasted away until at one time they feared he would not live. However, he eventually recovered and went on to become a sturdy, active child. Generally, his school reports were good, although at times he wouldn't try. His teachers recognized that he had plenty of ability, but at times lacked drive and was just plain lazy. When functioning at his best, he would be a straight "A" student. He made Eagle Scout at the age of fifteen, then volunteered to go into the service (Marine Corps) at the age of eighteen. Up until then, he had matured very well, but after discharge from the service in 1944, his mother said he had regressed, was unstable, restless, irresponsible, and had trouble making decisions as to a career.

His daughter Carol told me that he apparently found out about his adoption when he applied to go into the Marine Corps, as naturally they asked for a birth certificate. For some reason, his mother and father had never told him he was adopted. Carol said that in the early days of his marriage to Bernice, her mother, he disappeared for about three weeks, leaving no address or phone number where he could be contacted, and she wondered if perhaps he was searching for his real identity, his real parents, at that time. He also told Bernice that on no account was she to tell Carol that he was adopted. There is no way to assess what the

14

shock of this discovery did to him, and it's hard to understand the reason for all the secrecy, but no doubt adoption carried more of a stigma in those days than it does now, or his parents may have been sensitive about not being able to have a child of their own. In any event, I feel it could well have contributed to his instability and difficulty in adjusting back to civilian life. He seemed unable to find himself as a mature human being, completed high school two years after discharge from the service, and then tried some college courses. Although he had the mental ability to go through college, he didn't have the stability to follow through and would drop out or fail to complete his course work when under pressure. He finally chose the restaurant business, starting out as a busboy. Later on, in 1957, he completed two years of hotel-restaurant school in San Francisco, graduating with an A.A. degree. At this time, he really seemed to be on his way to solid achievement, was student president, and did very well in all his courses. His first job after leaving school was as assistant manager of the Press Club in San Francisco, and here again he received many compliments on his work.

He stayed in this position at the Press Club for about a year and a half, then left to start his own business—a tavern in San Francisco. This was run in partnership with another man, who apparently went bankrupt and left Dave solely responsible with a big financial burden. He did not again attempt a business on his own, but had various jobs as a maitre d', then switched to business courses at Armstrong Business College. From 1960 to 1963, he worked as a guard at San Quentin prison. When I met him in June of 1963, he had just dropped out of college, and shortly before, had been divorced from his third wife, Phyllis.

His first marriage to Bernice, in 1948, lasted about five years. He was apparently selfish, irresponsible, and immature and, as has been mentioned, would sometimes disappear for two or three weeks with no contact at all.

His second marriage, in 1952, to Dorothy Perry, lasted only three months, but in spite of that it was evidently one of the most meaningful of his relationships. I believe that he truly loved this woman and that even though they could not live together

15

happily, she was very special to him. He kept in touch with her for many years—took a real interest in her two children, Jim and Judy, as they grew up, and did all he could to be helpful. He had a signed photograph from Jim which said, "Thanks, Dave for being a friend." Dave has always been a compassionate, caring person, who would go overboard for those he loved. His loyalty to old friends and past associates was very strong.

His third marriage, in August of 1962, lasted about eight months. Phyllis was much younger—about twelve years or so. He told me that she spent money wildly, even charging her groceries, and that it nearly drove him around the bend. From another source I heard that he tried to dominate her, giving her little or no freedom and wouldn't allow her to drive or have a car of her own.

When I first met Dave, I knew he was cynical and bitter about his recent divorce and the fact that he felt he had made nothing of his life up till then. His father, George, and his uncle Jerry had both been very successful in their careers. George, an electrical engineer, was with the Pacific Gas & Electric Company for more than thirty years, ending up as vice president. Jerry was a prominent lawyer and on the Board of Regents at the University of California at Berkeley.

I married Dave because I cared what happened to him. It was a genuine feeling, even though I had ample warning as we got to know each other that he was not easy; prone to moods and inconsistency. Nevertheless, there was a basic honesty and frankness about him which was appealing. He made no attempt to put on a front or pretend he was anything he wasn't just to impress me. When I met his parents, I knew at once that this was a stable family. Strangely enough, the evening he invited me to go over to their home for dinner, I almost cancelled the whole thing—I had a strong impulse to run away, to break off the relationship. Reluctantly I went with him that evening, full of mixed feelings. My reward was meeting two delightful people who at once put me at ease and who, for the next twelve years, would play a major part in my life. They became a real family to me in every sense of the word.

16

And now, in September of 1975, this chapter of our lives was drawing to a close—a chapter in which Dave had lost the two most stable people in his life. Now he faced the future without the support of the two who I truly believe meant the most to him. He had relied on them and, I believe, had taken his sense of worth, his identity from them more heavily than perhaps any of us knew.

That second week of September, he was staying alone in their house on the last night before the remaining furniture would be moved out. He was sleeping in his mother's bedroom and had fallen asleep with the radio on, listening to a talk show. Some hours later, he didn't know what time it was, he awoke with the radio still on, and suddenly a vision of his mother appeared at the foot of the bed. She was radiant, smiling, and wearing a blue dress which had been one of her favorites. She looked just as real and alive as when he had last seen her. No words were spoken, but she stayed for what must have been several seconds, looking down at him as though in reassurance, then gradually faded. Dave was most emphatic that this was not a dream; he had been wide awake at the time. He called me the next evening to tell me about this, and I knew without a doubt that it was true. To me it was a very real sign that even though no longer with us physically, she knew and cared about his life and had come to him as a comfort and confirmation that she was very close in spirit. I felt it was a sign of special significance—perhaps to help us through the terrible times ahead, although at that time neither of us knew just what was to come.

The next three months, from September to December 1975, were not easy ones for us. Dave was restless, aimless, sometimes quite hostile for no apparent reason. He would also have spells of black depression and lethargy, when he would just lie on the sofa and sleep for several hours, sometimes for most of the day. Outwardly, it would appear that he was just lazy, but I sensed that it was more than that. Now without a job, he didn't seem able to develop other interests or hobbies. He didn't make any attempt to find himself work, and most frightening of all, nothing seemed to interest him. He worried constantly about when the estate would be wound up, although he'd been repeatedly told it would take about three months.

He went down to Oakland two or three times during this period, ostensibly to help Ruth with legal matters concerning the estate, but really I think he went mostly because of his old associations and because he felt completely at a loose end. One incident occurred which clearly showed that he was not functioning normally. We had a rental house close by that needed a new tenant. He was most suspicious of those who applied and turned most of them away with excuses that it wasn't ready yet or he had someone else waiting. Then a young couple applied, and rather reluctantly, he decided to rent to them. I left it up to him to make the arrangements, thinking it would be good for him to feel he was still useful and in charge of things. Then one Sunday when Dave was out, they knocked at the front door and said they had no key to the house. They wanted to get in and do some painting but could not telephone us as he had not given them his number. I hesitated, not knowing what he had told them. But how could he possibly rent the house if he didn't give the tenants a key? How could they make contact if he didn't give them his phone number? It was a risk, but I decided to go ahead and give them a key. Dave was furious with me. He didn't trust them, he said, but I was unable to reason with him, or point out that he should have arranged to go over to the house with them.

Most likely, he had told them verbally that they could have it, and had then forgotten what he'd said. As I remember, I also gave them our phone number, as it made no sense to me for tenants to deal with a landlord with no phone number. I am sure Dave felt totally inadequate to cope, and that was the reason for his suspicion; basically it was his own insecurity. He wanted to be able to handle it, and yet when it came to finalizing all the details, he had lost his grasp. What a tragedy. As it turned out, they never did rent the place. Dave was so suspicious that he convinced himself they weren't suitable, so told them he had changed his mind, they could not have the house after all. This was when they had already been in and started to paint, so they took the matter to a lawyer. Dave also got himself a lawyer. The

18

whole thing was unpleasant and unnecessary and finally cost a considerable sum in attorney's fees.

By contrast, my life was full of interest and fulfillment. I enjoyed my volunteer counseling twice a week; it got me out of the house and gave me something to think about other than Dave's problems. Often I felt guilty because life for me was so interesting, and I knew I had grown a lot through the experience of counseling such a wide variety of people. By comparison, what did he have to look forward to? About two weeks before Christmas 1975, his mother's estate was wound up, and he once more went down to Oakland to claim his share. Ruth told me that before he left her house to go to the airport, he was unable to find anything: wallet, glasses, airline ticket, and so on. When returning his rental car he got lost driving in Oakland, a town he had grown up in and known well since childhood.

On his return, he showed me the check he had received, and suggested that we should get some repairs and improvements done to the house. I heartily agreed, as there was much that needed doing. Dave was not handy around the house, so we always had to hire someone to do any repairs or maintenance that was necessary. Instead of following through on this suggestion, shortly afterwards he became heavily involved with his stockbroker, investing and making new stock purchases. In a way, it was a relief to me because it gave him something tangible to do, and for a time he seemed to take a new lease on life. He and Hugh became really friendly. Hugh gave him books on stock-market trends and the principles of investment; they often had lunch together and he spent many hours in Hugh's office. He talked about going into the stock market as a career, and if his mathematical ability and judgment had remained sound, this would have been a fulfilling avenue for him to take, both because of his liking for figures and for dealing with the public.

Shortly after receiving his share of the estate, he saw an advertisement in the paper for a post office and general store which was for sale down at the coast. It was at Tolovana Park, one of our favorite spots, and for a long time he had wanted to invest in some coast property. His idea was that Ruth and Nolan might

19

be interested in such an investment and we could run it jointly as a family business. He went down to see it on Christmas Eve, and liked it so well that he put down a deposit. I had told him before he left to be cautious—I wasn't sure that I wanted to move down there permanently, and having a business like this would tie us there for months on end unless we could get adequate help. However, he was so enthusiastic that he called Ruth and Nolan, persuading them to come up a week later to look it over. They made it clear that it was doubtful if they would want to invest in anything so far away from home; they wouldn't be able to help out much because of distance and at that time had no plans to move to Oregon.

We set out on New Year's Day, 1976, and had a pleasant drive down together, spending the night at a motel on the ocean front. It was a happy, relaxed evening, with an excellent dinner, followed by an enjoyable visit together in our motel room in front of a blazing fire. Next morning, we checked the property thoroughly with the broker who was handling the sale. It would have meant long working hours: 7:00 A.M. to 7:00 P.M. each day, and it would have been a major project for Dave and me to run it by ourselves. Fortunately, Nolan was astute enough to see that it would not be a really profitable operation, and tactfully persuaded Dave not to buy. I was thankful, yet felt sorry for him, as if only he had been capable, this might have been the kind of thing he would enjoy. Also I had visions of him starting out very enthusiastically and then losing interest. As things turned out, it was a blessing that we didn't go ahead with it.

A few days later we decided to trade in our VW which had been giving us some problems, and it seemed a good time to sell before it needed more expensive repairs.

For some time, Dave had been talking about getting an Audi Fox, and now that he had the money, it seemed a good time to do it. However, when it came to the point, he tried to back out. I persisted, reminding him that it was his idea, but he became defensive and tried to talk me out of it. I couldn't understand why, so I decided to hold him to it, and eventually he gave in, though very grudgingly. We set off in a silent, hostile atmosphere, stopped first at the bank to get the necessary funds and then on to the dealer.

During the time we negotiated and looked at different styles of cars, Dave was withdrawn, uncomfortable. He only spoke when asked a question, and then in an indifferent, offhand manner. I tried to draw him out as much as possible to make him feel it was as much his new car as mine, asking him what color he would like, trying not to push him into a hasty decision, and asking his opinion. Again, he was obviously having difficulty making up his mind. When it came time to drive the new car he seemed even more ill at ease. He did drive it, however, but seemed relieved when that was over. When the deal was closed, the salesman assumed that he would like to drive it home. Much to my surprise he said no, I could drive it. This was totally out of character—always when we were together, he liked to do the driving. As soon as that decision was made and we were on our way home, his mood changed completely. He was relaxed and all traces of resentment disappeared as though the whole incident had been wiped from his mind. I felt totally exhausted and drained, not understanding at all his attitude, yet thankful that we did finally get our new car despite his initial opposition.

It was now February of 1976 and he had been without a job for six months. He applied for a position as Motor Vehicle Representative with the state, and was helped in his application by a politician who was at that time running for Congress, and on whose campaign he had worked as a volunteer a couple of years before. The notice of interviews for the job came through in early March, and an appointment was made for him. Once again, he appeared to have new hope, which I shared. I longed so much for him to find his niche in life, humble though it might be at this stage, and admired the way he kept trying because I knew it was an effort for him and that his life in this respect had been an uphill grind all the way. He left for his interview in good spirits, and as always, I hoped for the best. He returned silent, not talking about it and I had to dig the details out. "I would have to learn to type," he said, and I knew by his attitude that things had not gone well. Apparently, there had been a panel

21

of four men who interviewed him, and he felt he had not come across well in his answers. The letter which came a few days later said: "We did not feel you were suitable for the heavy public contact which this job demands." Then he did something which I thought was so courageous. He wrote three letters of thanks to the people who had been instrumental in recommending him for the job, saying he had not been accepted but thanking them for their efforts on his behalf.

About a month later, he applied for a job as a nurse's aide in a local nursing home. He had been really down since the unsuccessful interview with the Motor Vehicle Department so I admired his courage in trying again. It was now almost a year since his mother had died, and I noticed that the shock and grief of that event seemed to be wearing off. Also perhaps he had the feeling that sometime there would have to be a break for the better in his fortunes. His interview with the director of nursing services went off well. They had a long talk and she must have sensed Dave's genuine compassion for older people because he got the job and started work in early April on the three-till-eleven shift. Almost at once there was a noticeable change for the better. So what if it was only as an aide? I admired him for being willing to start at the bottom, so to speak. In no way did I expect this to be a permanent job, but perhaps a stepping-stone back to better things.

He came home with enthusiastic accounts of the patients he had worked with—of the things they had said, of their reactions to him and to the other staff, of his impressions about the place. Once more, I felt promise; he appeared to be coming back into his own again after a long slump. Perhaps I was right that his strange behavior had been due to emotional shock following his parents' deaths so close to one another. Maybe now he was going to snap out of it. His work, though often consisting of menial tasks, seemed to be healing him because he felt useful and needed. Somehow he had surmounted the grief over his loss and was beginning to move on to a new constructive phase of life, a new beginning, perhaps built on the ashes of his sorrow.

I am sure that he established a genuine relationship with the six patients assigned to him, and that they responded to him with warmth and appreciation. To him I know they were real people, each with individual value, because of the way he spoke of them. The routine of our life together became purposeful again, and it gave me such pleasure to see him happy.

About a month after he started work, I met an acquaintance who asked me what he was doing now. I said, "He has a job as a nurse's aide at the convalescent hospital." An incredulous look crossed his face. I could tell that to this person such a job represented the dregs and was something to be hidden or glossed over if at all possible. I felt so proud of Dave that I didn't care what anyone thought. I admired him for taking this humble job and making it something special. What matter if the world thinks only of prestige, success, popularity, power, promotion? At that moment I knew the freedom that comes with being completely indifferent to what the world thinks. I was confident that at this point in time, the job was bringing him fulfillment in a way that could not be explained to those who think only in terms of worldly success. In May of 1976, Vinton, who was now working as an executive for a commercial real estate firm, asked Dave if he would like to take a test for a job as real estate salesman for that firm. Noticing his improvement, he was trying to encourage Dave to move on to work more suited to his training and talents. There were two written tests involved. One took about an hour and the other approximately thirty minutes. Vinton told me that Dave was able to complete the first, but had difficulty concentrating for long enough to finish it. When he came to the second test he just sat staring at the paper for a long time, apparently not knowing why he was there or what he should be doing. He didn't complete this test, and I remember he was down at Vinton's office for most of the day. When the results were analyzed, he had scored unusually high on the social-service aspects of the job, but his rating in the other sections was well below average. It showed that his practical day-to-day functioning was much below par. The day after, he was completely drained and exhausted, much more than one would normally expect.

Following this episode, Vinton took him aside one day over

23

lunch and suggested that he go to a doctor to find out what might be affecting him—causing the mental effort of a test to be so exhausting. He listened attentively to this advice, but didn't seem to think he needed medical help. After some thought he said, "All right, Mr. Vinton Green, if you think I should go and see a doctor, I will."

In early June, he went to our physician, Dr. Douglass, who gave him a thorough examination and an EEG. Neither of these tests showed anything conclusive, but Dr. Douglass recommended that he go to a neurologist for a more detailed examination. The neurologist made an appointment for him to have an EMI brain scan later that month. On the day he was due to go in for the scan, a telephone call from the hospital told us that the machine was out of order, so another appointment was made for July 8. During the time he was having these appointments with his doctor and neurologist, I noticed that he became more forgetful again. One day, the neurologist's office called to find out why he hadn't shown up for his appointment. I was surprised, thinking that they had finished all they needed to do, but apparently he was due that day for more tests, and had completely forgotten about it. Another time, while down at the hospital for further tests, he called me to make arrangements for us to meet later that day, as we had planned to have dinner together. He sounded very disconnected and hung up before we were even halfway through our conversation. This was his day off—a day that we had hoped to enjoy together, and now it was all disrupted.

There were again definite signs that he was not doing so well at work either; he was much less enthusiastic about the job, it seemed to be an effort to him, and he was often fearful of being left alone with a patient, especially if it was someone who needed to be lifted. He told me he was afraid of dropping a patient and being sued for it. One night he came home and told me he had "blanked out" on the floor. As he described it, he couldn't remember where he was, or what he was supposed to be doing. It sounded as though his mind had temporarily given up, perhaps from strain or pressure or an extra effort to concentrate. Even then, I didn't take this too seriously. No doubt I wanted to cling to the hope that he was getting better again—that this was just a temporary setback. I knew that it had shaken his confidence though, and had brought back his awareness that something was wrong. Also, the medical tests were weighing on him heavily, and toward the end of June, he decided to leave his job. I noticed that during his last ten days or so at the nursing home, his memory and recollection of what days he was supposed to be off were bad. He couldn't seem to get the dates straight in his head and was constantly checking with his supervisor.

Meanwhile, Ruth and Nolan had contacted us, saying they were going to come up for the Fourth of July weekend and stay a few extra days afterwards. It was a most welcome visit, but they were, of course, shocked to hear that Dave was once more without a job. They brought Susan, their second daughter, with them. She was seventeen and had always thought a lot of her Uncle Dave. I know it gave him a lift having them all there, and he made a special effort to take Susan out and make the visit fun for her.

We went to a picnic with Nolan's cousins—a large family gathering held at their farm in Yamhill county. It was a gorgeous summer day, with sun and shadow rippling over fields of wheat. Although Dave did his best to join in, I noticed he was sometimes ill at ease and really felt more comfortable by himself or with one or two of his own family. After lunch, Nolan took him off with some of the other men to work on a cottage that was being remodeled, and from all accounts this went off quite well. When it was time to go home, he asked me to drive, which was most unusual. After we had gone a few miles, he became agitated, thinking we were on the wrong road. "This isn't right," he kept saying; then, "Are you sure you're going the right way?" Evidently, he had not recognized where we were or remembered anything about the landmarks on the way as we drove out only a few hours before. It was not until we were in familiar territory that he calmed down, realizing we were close to home.

Another thing I noticed during that weekend was his inability to concentrate playing cards. We started a game of cribbage one evening, and each time Dave scored his hand he made mistakes, or had to be reminded when it was his turn to play. At first we thought he was fooling or in a facetious mood so we laughed, trying to pass it off as a joke. It was the worst thing we could have done, as he became moodily silent, withdrew from the game, and lay on the sofa for the rest of the evening hardly speaking, withdrawn into himself. Neither could we persuade him to go with us to a fireworks display at a neighbor's house close by. He preferred to stay at home with the two dogs.

The following Tuesday, Ruth and Nolan were going on down to Beverly Beach State Park with their camper, and invited us to go too. Dave, of course, had his appointment for the brain scan on July 8, but would be able to come down afterwards. He was not at all enthusiastic about the idea, and I really think he didn't want to go, so we didn't press him. I decided to go ahead, as always in the past he had never minded my going away for a few days without him. This was the decision I have regretted most of all during the past four years. If I had it to live over again I would have definitely stayed and gone with him to this appointment, as he really needed me then. Once again, I was trying to make light of the whole affair, and treat it as just another medical appointment. It is something I have felt guilty about for a long time. So often in life, the things that hurt the most are the times when we fall short in some essential inner value of our own, and it was certainly true in this case. Part of my excuse for not staying to go with him was that "it couldn't possibly be serious." Above all, I wanted to block out the reality that it could be serious.

As it turned out, he didn't go alone, as a good friend, Roy Frazier, went with him. But that does not excuse my failure to be with him at a crucial time—this is something I shall have to live with always.

2. *Diagnosis*

Two weeks went by, and we still had heard nothing from the doctor regarding the brain-scan results. So I called him; it must have been on or about July 21. He told me the news in a straightforward but sympathetic manner. "He has what we call Alzheimer's Disease." I had never heard of it, and had no idea what he meant. As he went on to explain what was happening to the brain, the whole thing felt more and more unreal; I was in a daze and so shocked that I really don't remember half of what he said, as I was trying to absorb the ghastly truth he was telling me. I do remember asking if Dave would be able to work, and he answered that possibly he could handle factory or assembly-line work—something that was mechanical or repetitive, where he would not have to use logic or reason or remember facts. The only way he would be able to remember as time went on would be by repetition, as the cells affecting memory—particularly short-term memory—were badly damaged.

The neurologist had the scan pictures in his office, so Dave would have to go back to him to get the full results, which he did the same week. This time I was more than ready to go with him, but he said no, he would go alone. Since I was not in on the interview with Dr. Bell, the neurologist, I don't know how he told Dave about the diagnosis, but neither one of us liked him. He had a flippant manner which perhaps disguised his own inability to break the news in a more compassionate way. No doubt our dislike of him was largely due to the fact that he was the bearer of such a terrible verdict. The scan showed that the left frontal lobe of Dave's brain was deteriorating fast; this was shown on the pictures by large blank spaces in between the cells. Dr. Bell's opinion was that since this damage was mostly due to a fluid buildup (hydrocephalus), a shunt inserted into the back of Dave's head might be helpful and would slow down the progress of the disease, although he admitted that there was no cure and no remission. In a shunt operation, a plastic tube is inserted at the base of the brain under the skin and remains there permanently, draining off fluid. It is invisible and apparently does not cause any discomfort. It is interesting that when we saw a second neurologist more than a year later, he said that no way would he have put a shunt in Dave's head. In his opinion, and in this particular case, it would have made no difference at all.

Dave's reaction to the shunt was negative, and I really didn't blame him as I felt the same way. It would have been an expensive, risky operation, a major trauma for both of us, and possibly no relief or improvement.

The remainder of that week was spent trying to adjust to the awful truth. It was a week when everything seemed blurred and unreal. We went through the motions of life, but underneath all the time was the dreadful pain and realization of what we had to face. Some time later, I had an interview alone with Dr. Bell. He showed me into his office, and then went out again to finish a conversation with another patient. When he came back, he left the door wide open, which struck me as unprofessional. Here we were about to discuss a terminal disease—something not only very personal, but highly painful emotionally. I was amazed that he had so little sensitivity or sense of privacy, so I got up and shut the door myself.

He stressed the importance of keeping Dave as busy as possible, questioned me about his hobbies, told me to quiz him on books he read to see how much he was retaining. He was doubtful that Dave should continue driving, and I knew he was concerned about safety because of slow reactions, forgetfulness in giving signals or remembering where to turn. During our interview, I noticed he was very evasive about many of my questions—I had made a list beforehand of the things I really needed to know. Either he did not know the answer, or was reluctant to give it if he did. Once he got completely off the point just to show that he had a knowledge of foreign countries, and again I felt a kind of disgust at his attitude. How could he be so flippant when the life and future of someone I loved was at stake? I came away with a feeling of horror—it's almost impossible to describe exactly the deep sense of tragedy I felt. I knew I would have to learn to live with this feeling somehow, that it wasn't going to go away. It's no good trying to comprehend the whole illness and the course it will take, anticipating the changes all at once. Shock and numbness are a blessing, otherwise we wouldn't be able to go on at all. But the raw truth is so devastating that it has to be absorbed a little at a time. It is enough just to live for the day, and truly those first days after the diagnosis didn't seem like life at all—perhaps this wasn't really happening to us— it was like being in a bad dream and looking in on ourselves from the outside.

A few days later, we went to a wedding. Roy's daughter, Sandy, was getting married and the ceremony was held at his house. It was a beautiful July evening, and the marriage took place outside on a patio overlooking the river. Dave and Roy had known each other well for some time and had also worked together in real estate several years before. It was noticeable that Dave kept himself apart most of the time. He was glad to see Roy and his brother, Earl, but stayed in the house during the whole ceremony, refusing to come outside. I stayed with him most of the time, and he appeared to enjoy the dinner afterwards. Earl noticed his withdrawn behavior and apparently said to Roy, "There's something wrong with Dave." At this point, neither of them had heard about the diagnosis.

The next day, Worth Bellamy called early in the morning. He had some business to do in the St. Helens area, and after he was finished would have some free time so he wanted to look over the Trojan nuclear plant. Would Dave like to go along? Dave accepted, and I was so thankful for anything that would tide us over our painful adjustment period, anything which confirmed that life was still enjoyable and worth living. I felt grateful to

Worth for being so considerate. He told me that so far as he was concerned, the day went off well. Dave seemed to be in excellent spirits and they talked freely all the way up to St. Helens; he was responsive and interested in hearing the latest news about the Real Estate Division, and on the surface there appeared to be nothing wrong with him at all. Even though they were together all day, Dave never did say anything about the diagnosis. When they returned that evening about five o'clock, Worth left him standing beside his car, still cheerful and to all appearances having thoroughly enjoyed their day out together.

As the evening wore on, and I had still heard nothing from him, I began to wonder what had happened. I thought perhaps they had decided to have dinner together and make a day of it. Worth and his wife had been good friends for several years and we had enjoyed many outings with them.

Ten o'clock came and I began to be really anxious. I called Worth. He said he and Dave had parted at about five that evening, so he should have been home long ago. I then told Worth about the diagnosis, expressing my concern. He said to check back with him if Dave hadn't returned by eleven. About half an hour later, he drove in and I was so thankful to hear the familiar sound of the car being driven into the garage. I had been sitting in bed reading, trying not to let my fears get the better of me. I didn't know what to expect. He was in a very depressed, hostile mood; defensive, because he doubtless knew that I would be worried. He told me he had had a few beers, but exactly how he had spent those five hours was not clear. I said, "I don't blame you at all for having a few drinks. I am sure I would have done the same under the circumstances."

It must have been a time of great desolation for him, fully aware now of the future that faced him. He must have dwelt at length on the implications of what the disease meant, plumbing the depths of a terrifying, dark precipice that had no apparent hope, no known solution and an indefinite, stark ending. I wonder how the soul endures at all in times like these, and once again I turn to Him who gave us the gift of life. Even in the worst that life hands to us, there is meaning. There has to be if we truly believe that He has won the victory, and that these terrible things will have only a temporary hold over us on this earth.

Shortly after the day out with Worth, Dave made plans to fly down and visit Jim Perry, his second wife's son, with whom he had had a close relationship when Jim was growing up. They lived in Los Angeles and Jim was now a successful dentist with a wife and two teenage daughters. When we talked to our travel agent about his ticket, he was very confused and needed constant reminders to get the facts straight in his head. I went out to pick up the ticket for him the day he was to leave. Wilda, our travel agent, when talking to him on the phone, had also noticed that something was wrong, so I poured out my heart to her. She was most supportive and understanding. She had always liked Dave, and it had been a congenial, happy relationship.

When I got back to the house, he was trying to finish up his packing. The suitcase was ready, so he told me to go on out and get the car started. I waited and waited. Ten minutes passed, then fifteen. I went in again to see what was happening. He was drifting around, looking for something, fumbling through his desk, then back into the bedroom, pulling drawers in and out, apparently losing track of what he was looking for. He had his keys, wallet, and glasses, so finally we went out and got in the car. Then he said, "I must go back and check something."

By this time, I was getting irritated and impatient. It was a hot day, and my anxiety was growing at all these delays. I was to learn later that this condition is aggravated by the heat. Finally, after about twenty minutes, we started and managed to get to the airport with minutes to spare before his plane left.

That weekend must have been a disaster. When I met Dave at the airport Monday evening, he came off the plane with a somber, ashen face. In fact, he looked right through me as he came down the ramp with a completely blank expression. "How did it go?" I asked.

"Not too good." While he went to pick up an evening paper, I went down to wait for the baggage to come off, expecting that he'd join me in a few minutes. The baggage from his flight came off and was claimed piece by piece, but no sign of his suitcase;

31

neither was there any sign of Dave. I began to feel apprehensive and went back up the escalator to see if I could find him, but he appeared to have vanished completely. I returned once more to the baggage-claim area, and walked the full length of that floor, but again with no result. After what must have been close to half an hour, an announcement came over the PA system. Would I please meet him at the United Airlines counter. When I got there, he seemed surprised: "Where on earth have you been?" he asked.

"Waiting for your baggage to come off," I replied.

"Oh, I don't have any baggage on this flight; I left in a hurry and it didn't get on the plane." With a sinking heart I went down with him to the parking lot. As we started for home, I tried to find out what sort of weekend he had had. The more he tried to explain the sequence of events, the more confused he became. Apparently, he had spent only one night with Jim and his wife. The next morning, they had had to leave early and left him alone for breakfast with a bowl of cereal. What a welcome! He then contacted Charlie and either rented a car, or flew to Carmel Valley. This was where he was most confused. He couldn't remember exactly how he had got there and kept contradicting himself. However, somehow or other, he did arrive at Charlie's. He could not make sense, either, of how they had spent the weekend, but whatever had happened, he was deeply upset, hurt, and troubled. The more I questioned him the angrier he became because he couldn't get his facts straight, and I never did get a clear picture of exactly what had happened. I remember feeling devastated. What nightmarish thing was happening so that he couldn't even answer simple questions about where he had been? He must have been badly hurt by Jim's casual treatment of him. It could have been that they, too, had noticed something was wrong, and had not been able to handle it, hence the excuse for having to leave early. Then Charlie, always excitable, apt to dramatize everything, couldn't have helped much. I had the impression that the time with Charlie was the last straw of a lost weekend. Eccentric and impulsive as he was, he must have contributed to Dave's confusion and may have made light of it, trying to laugh it off.

When we arrived home, Dave called Vinton, and I was amazed at how calm and normal he seemed in his conversation. I suppose the security of home and a talk with a close friend made the difference. There was no sign whatever of his anxiety of half an hour before. He asked me if I would like to talk to Vint, but I said no. I felt absolutely devastated and incapable of talking to anyone at that moment, trying to calm my own dread at what I'd just experienced. Dave was angry with me for not coming to the phone, and berated me for it afterwards. It was hard to explain that I really had nothing to say and I know that my grief might have been picked up by Vinton. It was no time to have to go into explanations.

The next morning, Dave was leaving to go to the United Airlines office to pick up his suitcase, which had been sent in on a later flight. Suddenly, he turned to me and said, "Where is the United Airlines office?" I couldn't believe what I'd heard. He had known that area like the back of his hand, and had passed that way countless times during the past twelve years. I swallowed my horror somehow and pulled myself together to try and give clear instructions. They were not well understood, and he got irritated at me for not being more explicit. However, he did find it, and I imagine that once he was on that street he recognized where he was, although he couldn't visualize it from a verbal description.

The rest of the day was a blur of pain, grief, and finally, extreme fatigue. During the past two days, I had had an example of the kind of things we were going to face. I wondered why neither of the doctors had given us some indication of what to expect, and how much worse these sort of episodes were going to be. I eventually got to a point where I couldn't feel any more and was thankful for that. How merciful are the times when our feelings are numbed. I am sure they are sent as a protection when we have reached the limits of endurance.

Life goes on somehow—I am amazed at the resilience of the human body, and how it snaps back after rest; how hope is always present somewhere in the background giving the incentive to move on, to keep trying.

In August, Ruth came to stay for a week, and it was a real help having her there in a time of great need. Dave went on one or two outings with us and took Ruth shopping one day, but otherwise was content to stay at home most of the time. Ruth invited him to go down and stay later in the month, and I felt it might be good for him to get away; he would be secure and in good hands with Ruth and her family, and the atmosphere would be peaceful.

About the eighteenth of August, he left in his red VW Dasher. I had no qualms because he appeared to have stabilized again, apart from some absent-mindedness. Once more, hope sprang; perhaps it wasn't as bad as it appeared. How one longs to bury the horror, the nightmare, not to have to face it. Acting on the doctor's instructions, it might be good for him to be as active as possible, because sooner or later there were going to be definite limits to what he could do, so why not live to the full while he had the capacity to do so. He still seemed confident and in control when driving, and it was one of the few things left he could still do to assert his independence. The morning he left, he seemed happy and carefree. He assured me he would call as soon as he got to Oakland.

It turned out to be an anxious week. Always in the past, he had called me when away from home, but the days went by and I heard nothing. He didn't appear at Ruth's. About the third evening, I contacted her, and we both had the same feeling—- that something was wrong. I also talked to Vint and expressed my concern. He said, "Dave is all right." I was too surprised to ask how he knew, but it was said with such confidence that I knew it was true. He did add, however, that if I wanted to pursue it further, he had contacts in California who would be willing to help in tracking Dave down. I thought of contacting Charlie, but knowing how he was apt to dramatize everything, decided against it. A couple of days later, Ruth called. She had heard from Rowena, a good neighbor of Dave's family who had lived next door to them for many years. He had dropped by quite unexpectedly one afternoon and stayed for about an hour, talking mostly about old times and his family. He had driven in at the back entrance and was standing outside the garage, gazing up at his old home, when Rowena came out and saw him. Surprised, yet delighted, she invited him in; said he had seemed relaxed, happy to see her, and she really didn't notice anything unusual in his behavior. She did notice, however, that when he left, he drove to the corner of Oakmont Avenue, stopped the car and stayed there for quite a while, as though undecided what to do. I wonder what went through his mind? Sadness, happy memories, remembrance of past associations? Perhaps he needed to say good-bye finally to this house which was no longer in his family. There could have been much nostalgia; a lost feeling, like being cut adrift and having no replacement. I feel he may have known instinctively that this was to be the last time he would ever see that house.

He stayed one night at a hotel in Oakland, but evidently spent most of his time driving, as he stayed at least two nights at motels on his way down and back again. I knew this from the receipts he brought home. He drove in quite unexpectedly one evening just in time for dinner, looking relaxed, suntanned, and glad to be home. He admitted to having been lost—said he had driven through a lot of hot, desolate country. From what he was able to tell me, he had left the freeway, possibly to get gas or a meal, and then was unable to find his way back, so wandered east into the Sacramento Valley instead of north, trying to get his bearings. He said he was thankful that the car kept on running, because at one point he was miles from anywhere and just kept going till he came to a motel. He had been fatigued by the drive; had forgotten what a long way it was.

After this adventure, Vinton urged me to get a second opinion. He felt impatient at our delay in getting to grips with the source of the trouble and trying to do something constructive. Perhaps there was more information that we didn't yet know.

In early September, I made an appointment with a second neurologist. However, the night before we were due to go in, Dave had car trouble. He was on his way home from Portland and had a flat tire, so I had to go and pick him up. It was late in the evening, so he left his car parked on the street, and would contact AAA in the morning. The phone calls to Triple A conflicted with our appointment which was at 9:00 A.M. so I had to call the office and cancel it, making an appointment for the following Friday at the same time. I can remember feeling so frustrated and angry as we left to pick up his car. It seemed as though fate were against us, and as though Dave was almost a pawn of fate in throwing up barriers to a better understanding of his illness. I flounced out of the house, slamming the door, furious with him for disrupting the day with his wretched car problems. He tried to calm me, but something inside resisted. I knew by now that we were in terribly deep water, so perhaps anger was a natural reaction. How could I express all my fears and dread to him? He who was already carrying his own awful burden.

In contrast to our hectic morning, that September day was crisp and clear with a definite hint of autumn in the air. Although I accepted Dave's explanation of a flat tire, on second thoughts, I am not convinced it was. He may have thought he had, but with his condition worsening, he could have exaggerated it, when really it was just a soft tire. It came home to me then how helpless he was about solving his own problems, if something as simple as this threw him. We never did get to that appointment. He flatly refused to go, and I felt too much compassion to push him any further. Besides, dragging him to a doctor against his will would have achieved nothing. Nevertheless, I sincerely would have liked a second opinion.

Still in the background was the feeling that this couldn't be real. *One day we'll wake up and find it's just been a bad dream. I am so terrified sometimes that I can't face my own fear. I don't know what may happen next, so I'll fill up time with compulsive housework, gardening, visits to friends, counseling, and encourage Dave to do as much as possible on his own. Blot out the reality, and act as if everything were normal.*

During that September two things happened. First, Dave became involved as a volunteer working for the state treasurer's political campaign. He worked in the office, answering the phone and delivering pamphlets, or doing whatever odd jobs were needed. This lasted several weeks, and was really a blessing, although I am not sure how much help he was to them. He told me one day he had been sent out to deliver some campaign literature and couldn't find the address where he was supposed to deliver it.

A benefit night at the theater was organized as a money-raising event, and he was involved in the planning of this. We had tickets to go, and he took me to dinner that evening. I remember we left the house much too early, and that instead of parking close to the restaurant, he couldn't seem to decide where to turn and went 'round in circles two or three times before he was able to park.

Just before the play was due to begin, he gave me my ticket and said, "Go on down to your seat; I'll join you in a minute." He stayed and talked to one of the campaign staff at the back of the theater, and by that time the lights had been lowered and the curtain went up. I looked back to see if he was coming, and saw him hovering in the aisle, apparently not knowing what to do. I waved to get his attention and he came on down to the row of seats behind where I was sitting. Thinking that perhaps he couldn't see too well, I motioned him to come around to the next row, but instead he started to climb over the seats from the back. Everyone looked around as he was causing a disturbance. He became embarrassed, turned around and pushed his way back to the aisle, then went to sit in the back of the theater on his own. Needless to say, the remainder of that evening was agony. It was impossible for me to concentrate on the play; even to sit through it took a lot of will power. After the first act, I went back and sat with him and the rest of the campaign staff. My heart and soul were with him, and of the impression he must have made on his coworkers. It was an immense relief when that evening was over—we had said our good-byes and were on the way home.

The second thing that month was the prospect of a trip to England. I had not seen my family now for six years, and the trip might just be a real boost for Dave. We made plans to leave the second week in October. Following his work on the political campaign, Dave went back to dealing with Hugh, his stockbroker. I was glad that he kept trying and the talk about stocks would surely keep him active. In the back of my mind however, was a nagging doubt that I hadn't expressed to anyone—that perhaps all this was risky. He could make a serious error in judgment, be talked into something against his will, or Hugh could take advantage of him. I did not know anything, really, about Hugh's integrity, although on the face of things he appeared to be a real friend to Dave. On his side, was the friendship genuine, or was he just cultivating the friendship in order to sell more and increase his commission?

As we finalized our plans for the trip to England, it became clear that Dave was not wholehearted about it. He knew, and so did I, that he might not be able to enjoy it as he had the previous time we were over in 1970. So I tried to leave it as open as possible, assuring him that he could cancel if he didn't feel up to it. Shortly before we left, Dave asked Vinton to go with him to the bank to check over the contents of his safe-deposit box. Vinton did so, and Dave seemed relieved and satisfied that everything was in order. However, a few days later, he contacted Vinton in a panic and said he had lost some important papers. He had been looking for them at home and couldn't find them. These were the same checks and other documents he had seen in the safe-deposit box only a few days before. Much of the time now he would go through his desk constantly, telling me he was clearing it out. In fact, clearing out his desk and other drawers seemed to be almost an obsession with him at this time, and he would spend hours doing it.

When we did get over to England, he didn't seem comfortable at all, and naturally for him the effects of jet lag took longer; it was also an effort for him to adjust to different surroundings. True, there were good moments. One highlight was the night we had dinner with a cousin of mine, Peter Hodgson, and his wife, Diana. There were seven of us that evening—my Aunt Joyce, Dave and myself, Peter and Diana, their son, Michael, and Diana's brother, Ben. They were all so warm and welcoming that Dave relaxed completely and was able to share in and appreciate all the jokes and reminiscences. They accepted him just as he was, paid him special attention, so I am sure he sensed this and responded accordingly. In the three weeks we were there, we had arranged to see as many of my relatives as possible, so travelling from house to house every few days was a necessity. Dave could not adapt to this and seemed fearful and ill at ease getting his bearings again in each house where we stayed. He seemed most at home with my sister, Helen, who was wonderfully kind and understanding, so we decided it was best to let him stay where he felt most comfortable. She told me that he was quite happy to stay in the house most of the day. Occasionally, he would take a walk in the village, or across to the church which was opposite Helen's cottage.

The hardest thing was knowing how to entertain him. When outings were arranged, he didn't seem able to enter in to what was going on, or lost interest quickly and asked when we were going home. We tried a wild-bird refuge, an autumn bazaar, a horse fair, and an old Roman campsite, with mixed success. When staying with a close friend of mine, Betty, and her husband, we took him to a pub lunch in a local town nearby. We tried to get him involved by making him order lunch for us, but even this was too much for him; he withdrew and asked us to do the ordering.

It was difficult getting him up in the mornings, and he would often take close to an hour shaving and dressing. If allowed to do so, he would be perfectly content sitting in front of the living-room fire all day unless someone dragged him out. Always, it was someone else who had to take the initiative. There were a couple of incidents which showed us that leaving him alone in a strange house might be dangerous. One night when at my sister's, he was the last one to go to bed and on his way to his room accidentally switched on the kitchen stove, thinking he was turning out the lights. In the middle of the night Helen's daughter woke up and smelled burning. It was fortunate that she did. On another occasion, at Betty's, he built a huge fire in the living room, forgot to put the screen in front, then wandered off upstairs. Her little dog, a West Highland terrier, was shut in the living room and Betty heard her howling about half an hour later. She came to see what had happened and found pieces of flaming wood already beginning to singe the carpet.

Dave had told me before leaving for England that he would like to spend some time in Holland as well, where he had enjoyed himself so much during our 1970 trip, but seeing him as helpless and dependent as he now was, I knew it was out of the question, so we discouraged him and the trip was cancelled. He was angry with me, and I really felt for him over this. It must have been intensely frustrating for him, being aware that he was not capable of handling this trip, and was terribly painful for me having to dictate what he should do or not do. I desperately wanted him to be able to do something on his own without having us in the background all the time, bossing, directing, doing what we thought was best for his own safety. It was such a fine line between his safety and his self-respect at this stage. He still wanted to assert his independence somehow, and kept on saying he would like to spend a few days in London before going home. Always, in the past he had liked to go off on his own to explore new places at his own pace and time, and I respected this need. Now, after much soul searching, I decided to let him go. We made a reservation for him at a comfortable London hotel. My sister put him on the train to London and then he got a taxi to his hotel. Apparently, it went off quite well and some older ladies staying in the hotel took him under their wing, invited him to tea, and entertained him. I think he got lost a time or two, but had the hotel address written down on a card, so was able to ask directions.

Again, this was a big risk to take, but I believe it paid off in terms of his self-esteem. He came home feeling at least he had achieved something on his own; it had proved that within certain limits he could still navigate by himself, even in a foreign country. I know too, that Divine Providence watched over him and protected him.

I had come home a few days early, and was glad of the time to catch up on the mail which had come in while we were gone. I had a shock when I discovered that he had overdrawn our joint checking account just before we left. He had purchased some stock and had instructed the broker to pay enough into our account to cover it, but there was a lapse of several days before this was done. This was totally out of character. He had always been meticulous in money matters and normally would have been appalled at the thought of an overdraft. Never before had he given me any cause to question his handling of our finances and I had always appreciated his integrity in this respect. Now I knew the time was at hand when he would no longer be able to handle money responsibly.

Dave's return from London was delayed four hours. I felt anxious, wondering how he would pass that time, and hoping he wouldn't wander off somewhere and miss the flight altogether. Also I knew it would mean extra fatigue for him, something he didn't need at this time. In spite of the twelve-hour journey, he arrived in remarkably good shape, recovered quickly the next day and seemed to attack life with some of his old zest. He brought a gift for me which he and Betty had chosen together. It was a King Edward VII souvenir plate, and more than ever I appreciated his thoughtfulness and his obvious pleasure in giving. He was able to talk about the last few days he had spent over there with pride and real gratitude for the way Betty and Helen had entertained him. He remembered many of the small kindnesses and things they had done which meant a lot to him. So the journey had been worthwhile; it had paid off in giving him a much-needed boost.

About a week after he got home, he got in touch with Roy—the friend who had gone to the scan appointment with him—and offered to help him move house. Roy and Mary were selling their home and moving back into an apartment. He spent the whole day with them and didn't get home till about six that evening. I was concerned in case it had been too long a day, yet glad that he could do something which made him feel useful. It was getting near the time when any small thing he could do to help his self-esteem would be valuable. It was often difficult to know just how much stamina he had. Some days, he would go and see Hugh, have lunch with him and spend most of the afternoon in his office, or would meet Vinton for lunch. This kind of stimulation was good and sometimes he would appear almost normal. One problem was that he had never had any hobbies except coin-collecting and racquetball, so getting him interested in something new at this stage was almost impossible. On the days when he had nothing planned, he would sit around the house, or wander in and out aimlessly, nearly driving me crazy. Spells of depression would alternate with times of being warm and affectionate toward me. I have mentioned his hostility earlier, but at the opposite end of the scale, on some occasions he was more open, more loving towards me than he had ever been before. It seemed that the defenses he had had over showing emotion openly were gradually disappearing, and in a way, this was one of the bonuses for me. Even a tragedy like this had compensation; that was why it was so important to live each day, each hour, to the fullest and make the most of the high spots when they came.

A few days before Thanksgiving 1976, Vinton took Dave out for the afternoon; at about 5:00 P.M. they were due at the airport to meet a friend of Vint's who was coming in to stay for a few days. They were sitting in the arrival lounge, chatting and watching the planes take off and land, when for a few moments Vint got up with his back to Dave and went to stand by the gate entrance as his friend's plane taxied in. He turned to say something to Dave but he was no longer there. He had disappeared into thin air in an unbelievably short space of time. Vinton explained to his friend that he had an emergency, then searched the airport lounge, the restrooms, the ticket counter, the main lobby, and finally went down the ramp into the parking lot. There he met Dave, coming back up the ramp. Vinton was understandably angry and also anxious at this extraordinary behavior. He really chewed Dave out, which would have been all right in normal circumstances. But here was someone who did not know the reasons for his actions or impulses—did not know what mysterious force guided him to wander off like this. I believe there must have been something in his mind which urged him to leave—a conviction that he was needed somewhere. He was surprised, apologetic, and when asked why he had left so suddenly, he answered: "They came to get me." He could not explain who "they" were, and it was never clear just what he meant. But now with the value of hindsight, I am fairly certain he had a hallucination.

When they got back to the house, Vinton came in ahead of

Dave and asked me if I realized how unsafe it was becoming to leave him alone now. This episode of wandering off could happen any time that he was not supervised. I understood what he was trying to tell me and knew deep down he was right. We were now entering a new phase of this downhill journey—one in which my role of protector would be even more marked, and his dependence would increase even more.

Vinton and Maria came to Thanksgiving dinner with us that year, and I remember Dave's confusion at the dinner table. He got mixed up with his knife and fork, and finally ended up with all the vegetable and gravy spoons on his plate. The sequence of helping himself to food and what to do with a dish afterwards was no longer clear to him.

It was at about this time too, that one day Vinton arranged to meet him for lunch at a familiar restaurant where they had often met in the past. They both took their own cars, and in his rear-view mirror Vint saw Dave turn on to a one-way street going the wrong way. Realizing what he had done, he pulled his car up on to the curb till he reached the end of that block, then disappeared completely for about forty minutes. He did eventually make it to the restaurant, and was apparently none the worse, but the shock of this must have made him forget for the time being where he was, so he probably got lost trying to find his way back. It is interesting that when he told me about this experience, he tried to treat the whole thing as a joke, and it occurred to me that perhaps his sense of danger might be impaired if he didn't take something like this seriously.

On one occasion, he brought home a dead cat he had found lying in the road, and buried it in the garden. It was not buried deeply enough, however, and our dogs dug up the carcass, which then had to be reburied, this time at a safe level. His preoccupation with dead or wounded animals seemed to take on a morbid, unhealthy aspect at this time.

December came, and one Saturday afternoon he became very hostile toward me. He was verbally abusive and I could do nothing right, so to get away for a while, I took the two dogs for a long walk. It was a raw, foggy day and I had nothing on my head. That evening, as I was getting dinner, I started to have an acute earache in my right ear. It would come and go with knife-like stabs. The pain continued off and on through that weekend, so on Monday I called my doctor only to hear that he was fully booked for the next ten days. I went to the out-patient clinic of a local hospital where I saw a doctor who gave me some drops to use at regular intervals, but he didn't seem able to diagnose it. Three days later, the pain decreased, but the right side of my face gradually started to go numb, and the following weekend I had no movement in that side of my face. Eventually, I went to an ear specialist who diagnosed it as a mild case of Bell's Palsy. He told me it would clear up of itself in time—to keep the right side of my face moving as much as possible, and to keep the ear covered in cold weather. It did slowly improve and was normal again about a month later, but I still have an uneven right side—the eyelid is weak and the right sinus more susceptible to irritation.

Although being out in the cold must have started the whole thing, I know that the strain of dealing with Dave's behavior must have played a major part in the severity of this. For quite a while afterwards, the right eye would run when exposed to the cold. Dave overcame his hostility and was genuinely sympathetic to my plight, but he didn't seem to take in for any length of time what was happening.

Soon after Christmas, he came down with a heavy cold and cough which he didn't seem able to shake off. It hung on for at least two weeks and it was obvious that he was weakened by it and unable to bounce back with his old resilience. At this time, he would often have bouts of depression, or would pace up and down the room for hours at a time. There would be angry outbursts at me—most often when I was trying to help him and show my sympathy. I felt so sorry for him as I knew he felt rotten physically as well as mentally, but having to bear abuse when one is trying to help—to have kindly gestures thrown back in anger—is one of the hardest things to bear. I wonder just where his mind was at times like these. It may be that his perception of my intent toward him was flawed, or perhaps he felt resentment because he knew he was slipping and my attentiveness just confirmed it all the more.

January, 1977 dawned cold and dry. It was the year of the winter drought in Oregon. We had not had anything near our normal winter rainfall; each day was clear and frosty and we often had fantastic sunrises, some of the most spectacular I have ever seen. Although we desperately needed rain, there was a kind of tranquility about those serene winter days as though time was standing still, refreshing our lives with something completely different from normal. On New Year's Day, we had a light dusting of snow, but it soon vanished to be replaced by the calm, dry weather that was now becoming so familiar.

As usual, during the first week of the month, the bills came in. I brought these to Dave's attention and said I had noticed that the balance in our checking account was getting low. This brought forth an outburst. "I am not going to pay any more bills," he raged. "Why should I? I don't have to pay them and you're not going to tell me what I should do. If you need more money, why don't you go out and get a job?" He was so furious, so impossible to deal with at that moment, that I felt the best thing I could do was to go out for a while and just drop the whole thing. I felt cold and sick inside, and wanted so much to run away. I remember telling myself I would have to leave, I couldn't possibly go on living with him if we couldn't even communicate about everyday matters such as bills anymore. Eventually, I went home praying for a better situation, and found he had calmed down and seemed to have forgotten the whole incident. I didn't say any more about it; just sat down and wrote the checks trusting that there would be enough money to get us through the end of the month. Another problem was that he would take the income from his stocks and reinvest it again, thereby leaving little or no money for living expenses. Sometimes, he would leave checks lying around for weeks without depositing them in the bank. On more than one occasion, I took his income checks and deposited them without saying anything, terrified that he might lose them or accidentally tear them up. I felt guilty about doing this—that I was cheating him—and yet it seemed the only way I could

45

handle this without an angry confrontation.

At one time earlier on, when his reasoning ability was better, I had tried to point out as tactfully as I could that this policy of reinvesting all his income didn't make sense now that he had no job. I tried to tell him that there were repairs that needed doing around the house, help with keeping up the garden, as well as the routine bills and medical expenses, but I met a blank wall of resistance. He was not angry, just stubborn and didn't seem able to grasp what I was trying to tell him. I knew there was no point pursuing it any further, because his self-image was damaged enough, not being capable of working anymore, and my suggestions might be construed as criticism in a very sensitive area. I knew then that we had to get help over money matters, since he would not accept my handling of his affairs.

After the difficulty I had with him over paying bills, I went to a lawyer to find out what could be done about money matters in a case like this. He explained that a conservatorship might be the answer. Someone who would be responsible for handling his finances, though not actually a personal guardian, since I, as his wife, fulfilled that role. If he was not willing to accept a conservator, the court would have to certify him as legally incompetent before anyone could be appointed. What a prospect! I had now entered a phase where I had to do things behind his back for his own safety. This was terribly painful, and I felt like a traitor.

Also, during this month I knew that I was going to need help and support such as I had never needed before. One morning, I went to the pastor of my church and poured out the whole story. After the first few minutes, I broke down and cried through most of the remainder of our talk. He told me that there was a prayer group which met weekly on Thursday mornings and he would tell them about our crisis. The following Thursday, I joined that group. I remember so well their immense compassion and understanding. I had never, up till this time, learned how to pray out loud. All I could do that day was to blurt out my grief and cry again. They gathered around and laid their hands on me, accepting my tears, my sorrow, without question. It was the beginning of a new growth spiritually for me. I had to learn to take my eyes off our terrible problem and trust solely in God. It was to be my one lifeline during the months and years to come.

It is important to say at this point that since the diagnosis six months before, both Gwen and I had attended services of healing two or three times to pray for him. The morning after our dreadful confrontation about bills, Vinton had taken him to the same service, which was held in the chapel of Good Samaritan Hospital. It may seem strange that I did not go too on this occasion, but I was so bruised and injured by the events of the day before, that I just couldn't face it. Many others who were aware of the situation were also praying, but now I had to face the fact that these prayers might not be answered in the way we would have hoped. He was not improving.

As the month wore on, I noticed that he seemed more and more depressed and listless. Meanwhile, in a purse which I had not used for some time, I found a card. On it was the name of a Chinese doctor who practiced acupuncture. The card had been given to me by a client at William Temple House, the agency where I did volunteer counseling. This client had been to see Dr. Hung for a back problem which was very painful and had been completely relieved of his pain to the point where he no longer needed medication. I remember when he gave me the card he said: "If you ever need medical help, go to him; I really recommend him."

Not long afterwards I called Dr. Hung's office and asked if acupuncture had ever been used for brain disease. He said that he had not personally treated anyone with Alzheimer's Disease, and told me it was very important that Dave be willing to come in for a consultation before he could decide whether to treat him or not.

After I finished my conversation with the doctor, I went out into the living room. Dave was standing with his back to me, staring out of the window, his hands in his pockets, apparently in a pensive mood. Cautiously, I brought up the suggestion of acupuncture. We had been given no hope by conventional medicine, so what had we to lose? I tried to be as optimistic as possible, as positive as I could be. Would he at least go for a consultation? Then, if he decided he didn't want to have treatment, I wouldn't force him. Somewhat reluctantly, he agreed. I didn't know whether he would still feel the same when it was time to go for our appointment the following Tuesday, but I was encouraged by the fact that at least he had not put up any major resistance. In my heart, hope sprang again. Perhaps this was the answer, the miracle, we had prayed for.

3. *Acceptance*

The farther I have gone along this road of crisis, the more I realize that for several years beforehand I was being prepared to meet it and to live it. This preparation came in the form of experiences in counseling, seeking to understand and enlighten those traveling through their own deep waters—so often it was they who taught me more about myself—the things that they were going through, I had experienced myself, so they reflected back to me a part of myself as I identified with their suffering and tried to find a constructive solution. I came to learn that if we are open, we never stop growing and learning; age is immaterial so long as the desire to move on is still there; to be challenged by new ways of responding to whatever life brings.

Next, I was prepared by the friends who came into my life, the books I read, the sermons I listened to. Suddenly, my faith came alive in a way that was real and exciting, in a way I had never known before. A foundation was being laid during the early '70's on which I would build, and without knowing it, I was putting down deep roots into this foundation which would ultimately hold me steady when the storms came.

Perhaps the greatest single source of spiritual strength came from Dave's mother. Her belief was not in word only, but in example. She lived what she believed, and this became clearer to me as time went on. Even now, almost six years after her death, I can still look back and see what her example did in both of our lives. I know that she was used as an instrument to deepen our faith, to make it real. And so, we moved into 1976 facing disaster, although unaware, mercifully so, what the year would bring.

When the news of our tragedy was presented that July day, the first reaction was shock, extreme grief, and dread of what the diagnosis implied. Over the next few weeks, there was a measure of disbelief, of unreality. After the initial shock had worn off to some extent, I denied reality—perhaps the diagnosis was wrong, perhaps the disease wouldn't progress. Always with me was the hope that God would heal him; that there would be a miracle. Therefore, I dragged my feet about getting a second opinion. It was so much easier to remain with the hope that he would be healed than struggle with the emotional trauma of a second opinion. What if it was the same as the first diagnosis? I don't think either of us could have faced that all at once. The stark truth is much too hard to absorb completely, so acceptance comes only by degrees and cannot be forced. I am sure that each one of us has a different capacity and a different pace in learning to accept. It seemed to me that there were set stages to be gone through, and these should not, indeed could not be hurried.

As time went on, I gradually began to accept his limitations. The doctor had told me that he would in all probability not be able to work any more, but if he did, only mechanical or repetitive work would be suitable. So the next stage, and probably the hardest of all, was learning to live one day at a time. The future is unknown and it doesn't bear thinking about. This is where my faith was first put to the test—the first lesson in living one day at a time. So easy to say, so hard to do in practice.

In this disease, progress is usually so slow in the early stages that perhaps acceptance is easier because it is more gradual. In between lapses, behavior often returns almost to normal. The worst times were those when he would become hostile to me for no apparent reason, but this could have been not only a symptom, but an expression of his own inner turmoil, grief, and despair over what was happening. This hostility took the form of resenting that he had to be reminded where things were and my bossiness in trying to direct him or dissuade him, as the case might be. He must have gone through hell realizing that he was getting more dependent on me all the time, he who had always been so independent, and for me it was tragic to watch this and a major burden to be forced unwillingly into the role of dominance. Often, I would hear myself telling him what to do, or having to correct him, and there were many times when I hated myself. But what alternative was there? I was responsible for his safety, his day-to-day life, for making it run as smoothly as could be expected in such circumstances. I had to continually try new ways of communication as his personality changed and to adapt to these changes; to be aware of his moods which also changed rapidly because of forgetfulness or a short attention span; to try and keep my own head above water; to deal with my own intense sorrow and exhaustion at times; to fight off the blackness of dread concerning the future, his future, our future—where would it all end? How can we possibly live through this? What will happen when it gets so bad that I can't handle him at home any more?

I came to learn by experience that God gives us sufficient strength for whatever may be needed. At times, he seemed to throw a protective veil around my feelings so that I was numb and therefore immune to happenings which would otherwise have overwhelmed me. By shutting off my feelings, he gave me freedom to act in a matter-of-fact way, to be constructive, to get on with the business of living, for life must go on. I also learned that when I come to the end of myself, as I did so often during those terrible four years, the only thing left and the one thing that matters, is my relationship with Him; there is really nothing else. He is the only lasting source of comfort, peace, and strength. He will walk every precipice we meet in our lives with us, if we call on Him. Usually, it is the last thing we would choose ourselves, but He can turn it into growth, maturity, and victory. Victory over fear, over death, over the unknown future. That is not to say we don't suffer physically or emotionally. We do, for we were never promised freedom from sorrow in this life. But there is the inner assurance that all this has been overcome because we have for our guide the creator of the universe—He who is all-knowing, all-seeing, everywhere present—a God of compassion and understanding who has travelled the same road in human form and

51

identifies with every suffering we shall have to face.

No matter how desperate the journey, then, we are not alone. The absence of joy does not mean the absence of God, for he is just as real in our pain as he is in our joy, even though we may not always feel his presence. Kahlil Gibran, writing in *The Prophet* says: "And could you keep your heart in wonder at the daily miracles of your life, your pain would not seem less wondrous than your joy; and you would accept the seasons of your heart, even as you have always accepted the seasons that pass over your fields. And you would watch with serenity through the winters of your grief."

A major problem of acceptance was the fact that our prayers for healing had not been answered, which brought up the question asked countless times: "Why does God allow this to happen? Why does he not respond? It is surely not his will to punish in this way, so how do I deal with that?"

The ideas which I express now are not based on fact; they are pure speculation and what I feel may be the truth so far as Dave was concerned. I feel perhaps that he had no real will to go on—to fight back—to live. True, the diagnosis was hopeless. But perhaps it was something which, subconsciously, he wished would happen. I don't mean in such a terrible way. But something which would take all responsibility from him, so that he would no longer have to cope with everyday life. He had had so many blows in his life, and after both his parents died, this may have been the last straw. So, in a sense, he may have brought it on himself. The sum total of all his failures, disappointments, and setbacks may just have triggered this disease. Perhaps it had been latent within him for some time—possibly even a result of some brain damage sustained at birth when he was so tragically abandoned as a baby. Whatever the reason, I believe his will may have been involved, that in some way he allowed it to happen. His mind, instead of working constructively for him, worked against him. How subtle and infinitely complex is the human brain.

If my speculations are true, then, he was working against the natural laws of healing by consciously or subconsciously wishing to withdraw from the struggle. After we had had the diagnosis, he rarely talked about it or his feelings. Perhaps it was altogether too much for him to handle, to verbalize, and as stated in a previous chapter, he was never one to open up easily. I could only tell how he was feeling by his expression or attitude. To be honest, it would have been hard for me to talk to him about it myself, as my sorrow and concern for him would have been overwhelming.

However, I am convinced it is never God's will that anyone should suffer through a terminal disease. But we live in an imperfect world, where disease and sin abound, so we are all subject and vulnerable to these afflictions. True, there are cases of miraculous, unexplained healing from time to time, so why not in Dave's case? It's too big a question for me to answer. I do know, though, that God's presence has been with us all through this wilderness; that he has revealed himself in answered prayer by giving me strength and peace and assurance. I don't know what his purpose is in Dave's case, and even if I did, would probably not understand. So I have to accept my human limitations, trusting, indeed knowing that He is in charge and in his own way and time will bring Dave's life to perfection and wholeness. Life on this earth is a very short, but important chapter of our existence. We have been promised that "the sufferings of this present time are not worthy to be compared with the glory which shall be revealed in us." If this is true, we don't need to ask questions about the things we don't understand in this life; it is enough to know that this promise is real.

4. *There Has to Be an Answer*

And so, the morning came for our consultation with Dr. Sian Ming Hung. As we drove to his office, I prayed that Dave would remain open, willing to follow through, and wouldn't suddenly change his mind and refuse to go. If he did, there was really nothing I could do, as forcing him against his will would just make matters worse.

Dr. Hung was courteous, interested, and expert at putting us at ease. He seemed to be trying to evaluate Dave not only as a case history, but as a whole person. I noticed that while he was talking, he held Dave's wrist for several seconds, not only to give reassurance, but also to take his pulse. He explained how acupuncture worked and what he would try to do if he accepted him as a patient. His purpose would be to try and stimulate parts of the brain that were still normal to take over some of the functions now impaired because of damage or loss of brain cells. The treatment with acupuncture needles would stimulate functional improvement in nerve transmission to the brain. It would improve the function of nerves still intact, but could not reverse the deterioration of the neurons already lost.

At the end of our consultation, Dr. Hung hesitated quite a while, pondering whether to accept Dave as a patient or not. I believe that he was trying to assess whether Dave really wanted to get well. Even though the diagnosis held out no hope, was he the kind of patient who had the will to try against heavy odds, to fight back?

Dr. Hung later explained to me that he was hesitant to treat Dave because he knew well that Alzheimer's Disease is irreversible. The diagnosis is always so poor that there is a question as to whether there will be any beneficial results. Before treating a patient, he always takes into account whether the results will be positive; in this case it was most important to be reasonably confident that Dave would derive at least some benefit from acupuncture. In his evaluation, he took into account the fact that Dave was physically healthy, not addicted to drugs or alcohol, and the fact that we came together as a family, genuinely seeking help; he could see that we were desperate, and trying to find some answer to this awesome dilemma. These factors made him decide to go ahead and accept Dave. During that consultation, he gained our confidence with his thorough, yet warm approach. It was important that I, as the wife, come in with Dave and support him in his treatment. "To me, husband and wife are one," he said. I could tell that Dave liked him and my hopes began to rise once again. We made an appointment for the following Tuesday for the first acupuncture treatment.

When that morning came, I reminded Dave that this was the day for his first treatment. For a long time now, he had not been able to remember what day of the week it was, and of course had completely forgotten about the appointment. It must have come as a shock to him because he was very uncooperative and flatly refused to go. He liked Dr. Hung well enough, but didn't like the part of town his office was in, neither did he like the other patients he had seen there. True, Dr. Hung treated all kinds, and some of his patients were those who lived on Skid Row. The office was unpretentious, but that had nothing to do with the quality of treatment. I felt despair rise within me; the one chance we might have for some help was slipping away. If he persisted, I could not force him. We ate breakfast and I got dressed. Meanwhile, Dave sat in the living room, still rebellious, so I knew it would be useless to say any more unless his mood changed. With about half an hour left before we were due to leave, I said, "If you don't want to go, I'll go myself for a consultation." There followed about fifteen minutes of indecision, after which he surprisingly gave in, although in an ill-tempered, taciturn mood.

All the way to the office, I knew we were walking on thin ice—at any moment he might change his mind again, refuse to go in when we got there, or insist on leaving before his treatment. Not only was he reluctant to try again, but perhaps resented the fact that the treatment had been my idea—just one more indication that he was losing the ability to make his own decisions and be independent.

Once again, Dr. Hung skillfully put him at ease. He had a kindly, unhurried manner. He inserted a needle behind each ear, one in his forehead between the eyes, one in each wrist and one in each leg, midway between the knee and ankle. He told Dave to lie still and relax while the needles were in. The needles are fine, like hairs, and usually painless, although I noticed that Dave flinched when they were inserted behind his ears. Their function is to set up impulses into the central nervous system, releasing the body's own morphine-like substance, endorphin. The endorphin in turn releases the body's hormones to promote healing, retard aging, relieve nerve tension, restore organ function, and improve the body's defenses.

After the needles were inserted, Dr. Hung left them in for about twenty minutes, while he went to see another patient. Periodically, he would come back and twirl the ends of the needles. I sat with Dave during this time and could hardly belive that finally I had got him to accept this treatment; it was a miracle that he had been willing to come in after so much intense opposition. I felt immense relief and thankfulness; it seemed as though a major hurdle were behind us.

Following the treatment, Dave perspired heavily as was shown by the sheet on his couch; it was drenched with sweat, and Dr. Hung told me that his nervous system was badly out of shape. He should take it easy for the next twenty-four hours. Thus began a series of weekly treatments which were to continue until July of that year. Usually, they were on Tuesday afternoons. After the first couple of visits, Dave's suspicion and resistance gradually lessened; he began to really trust Dr. Hung and realized he was being helped.

About three weeks after our first treatment, we were having dinner with Vinton and Maria one evening. Suddenly, Dave began to perk up, took an intelligent interest in the conversation, and showed his sense of humor once again. On our next visit to Dr. Hung's office, we passed on this welcome news, and he gave the "thumbs up" sign. This was the first indication that the treatments were beginning to have results. The restoration of his sense of humor was a very positive signal of some return of functioning in a more normal way. That day Dr. Hung predicted that if the improvement continued, we could expect as good as a 50 percent remission, and we went home floating on air. Now the tide had turned, or so it seemed, and it felt so wonderful to have a definite improvement to look forward to. Our struggle to find an answer had paid off. Painful and difficult though it had been to get him to go for treatment, now we were reaping the benefits of having tried; we had not just accepted the inevitable, we were fighting back with a good chance.

Although in some ways Dave was easier to deal with at home, the problem of financial matters still remained, and this was an area where it was dangerous and risky to leave him on his own. Much as I hated to have to pry into his affairs, it was essential, and we had some really bad scenes over money. Whenever I would ask for housekeeping money, he would either say he didn't have any (which was totally untrue), or tell me to go and get a job. It was often frightening to deal with him, because there was a completely blind spot where my needs were concerned. I dreaded the first week of each month when the bills came in, as I knew we would go through the usual hassle, generally ending up in an angry, abusive confrontation. It's hard to describe, but I had a sense of hopelessness, of my requests not being understood because the part of his mind which would normally respond to something like this was just not there any more; the ability to understand my needs and my fears and listen to them was gone. Sometimes, after he had behaved in an impossible manner, he would try and make it up to me by taking me out to dinner. I am sure that he had no idea just how difficult he was, and no doubt thought that I was the one who was demanding.

In early February, I had closed our joint account and opened a separate account in my own name. I hated having to do this, but it was the only safe course to take. He responded by opening a checking account of his own at a different branch. He was still dealing with Hugh, his stockbroker, but I noticed that now there was an increasing reluctance to venture into new stock purchases, probably because his understanding and comprehension of financial deals was slowly getting worse all the time, so he felt insecure.

However, Hugh called the house one day when Dave was out, told me that he had some promising new stock, and would like to talk to Dave about it. When I told him, he seemed unenthusiastic, then forgot to call Hugh back, so I hoped the matter would be dropped. It is important to say here that about two months before, I had talked to Hugh myself, telling him that Dave had a neurological problem which affected his memory. I didn't go into any detail, but warned him of possible lapses or inconsistencies in Dave's behavior and to be on the lookout for these. It was really an appeal to Hugh's integrity—I had hoped so much that he was a real friend, and having had this warning, would react accordingly. But he persisted in calling and trying to pressure Dave into this purchase, which involved a considerable sum of money. Dave didn't seem able to deal firmly with Hugh, and instead of giving a definite no, he would hedge, thereby laying himself open to more pressure. Finally, I weighed in heavily and said, "When Hugh calls again, just tell him you're not interested." He did this, saying he would not be interested in further stock purchases for the time being.

Our loyal friend Vinton had been aware for some time of the difficulty over finances, and one day he was able to put it to Dave as tactfully as he could. He could see that he was going to need someone to help in this area, and did he have anyone in mind? Dave answered, "There's only one person I would trust to handle my affairs, and that's Vinton Green." He told me about this conversation, and I felt so thankful that this was a real possibility. I wanted to go ahead at once, but Dave, sensing my eagerness, backed off and the matter was delayed for almost two more months. Meanwhile, it came forcibly to our attention just how incapable he was of handling his own bank account. One day he received his monthly statement which showed that he was overdrawn and one of his checks had bounced. He was furious; he couldn't understand how this could have happened. Someone else must have written a check on his account. He stormed out of the house and I remember feeling nauseated because I knew it was impossible to present the truth to him. It no longer registered and he could not grasp the connection between his own responsibility and the outcome of his actions. On this occasion, I just felt he'd have to handle this himself; maybe it would get through somehow even in his confused state that he needed help. Perhaps it was a good thing this had happened.

The acupuncture treatments continued on a weekly basis, and about mid-April he was able to drive himself down to the doctor's office, giving me a much-needed respite from this task. Dr. Hung told me that that day, he behaved almost normally, acting in a way one would expect of a mature man of his age. However, he warned me that as Dave improved, he would challenge me more at home as he felt himself becoming stronger and more capable. It would be the kind of behavior one might expect from a teenager testing a parent—mentally now he was on a par with someone of that age.

Indeed this was true, for shortly afterwards we had a major blow-up—I forget exactly what caused it—perhaps my extreme weariness and lack of patience at this time because of the long strain we had been under; also the question of Vinton taking over management of his money was still hanging in the balance. At any rate, he said, "This marriage isn't going anywhere, Claire, why don't we get a separation?" This was the last straw and I felt more desperate that day than I had for months. It came at a time when he had begun to improve so that he was noticeably more independent and outgoing, and I had longed so much for better things in our relationship. I remember that I did almost leave him. I went so far as to telephone and reserve an apartment. It would have been a relief to solve the problem once and for all by running away from it. I could have justified it by saying that this was what he had asked for, and yet . . . deep down I knew this was not the solution.

That night in despair I went over to talk to a neighbor, Delores Hansen. As I look back I can see that always in time of need, there was someone to talk to, provision was always made for support when I was at the end of my rope. Delores filled just such a need that night. We talked for almost three hours and during that time she made me see, in a compassionate way, what a mistake it would be to leave him. As we talked, sharing some deep feelings in an honest, open way, I felt my strength returning. I knew she was right when she pointed out that I would create a worse hell for myself if I did run away, because my conscience would give me no peace and I would have to live with that for the rest of my life. With great wisdom and perception she told me that he really needed me now, even though he pretended otherwise. I had to see beyond the surface talk of separation, to ignore this and remain stable no matter what the cost. Knowing that Delores was close by and one to whom I could turn in a crisis changed the whole picture. The gratitude I felt for her kindness in listening and just being there at this crucial time is something I shall remember always. I went home that night refreshed, feeling able to face the next day with whatever it might bring.

Toward the end of April, Dave was finally persuaded to accept Vinton's offer of help as a conservator. Vinton himself had done much soul-searching before deciding to take this on. He knew he would have to face difficulties in handling an extremely sensitive and personal area of Dave's life, and had asked himself whether their friendship demanded that he be "his brother's keeper" in this respect. It might mean the loss of the friendship altogether, for undoubtedly there would be things which would be unpleasant and painful for both of them. He would slowly and gently have to take the responsibility from Dave's hands, while still showing him the warmth and respect of a friend. He was well aware of Dave's changing moods so he would need exceptional patience and tact to deal with these, and also with a very natural suspicion and opposition on Dave's part. In effect, it involved taking away a vital part of his self-esteem, although we hoped so much it would only be a temporary measure and that eventually, if he improved sufficiently, responsibility for his own affairs would be handed back to him.

Our first step was a visit to the bank to go over the contents of the safe deposit box. In fact, there were two boxes at different branches of the same bank. As we checked off the items and made a list, Dave became increasingly restless, and when it came to checking over envelopes containing legal documents he was noticeably on edge. Once he told Vinton an emphatic *no,* he was not to open that envelope. It was the one containing his adoption papers. Vinton respected this and was most tactful all through that long session.

This was to be the first of many visits to the bank, for there were a number of things to be listed, and also savings accounts to be closed. Things did not always go smoothly, and Vinton had to walk a tightrope often when dealing with delicate matters in which Dave had always used his own judgment. Most often, it involved decisions as to how money should be invested, or what kind of an account should be set up. On many occasions, Dave was balky and understandably so, and would respond: "I'll do it my way," when trying to assert himself. If we had taken one wrong step that would have upset him, we could not have forced him to accept Vint's authority over his affairs, so this again was another precipice. Legally, we had no right to force him, if he flatly refused to go along with Vint's suggestions.

The conservatorship had to be set up through the court and the appointment of Vinton as conservator approved legally. First of all, we had to make a complete inventory of all property and stocks in Dave's name, so there were frequent visits both to the bank and to an attorney during those first weeks of May. When the inventory was complete, the whole matter had to be presented to the court for their approval. All this took about a couple of months, so during that time Dave had to be willing to go to the bank with Vinton to transfer funds from his savings to a joint checking account to meet our monthly expenses. I well remember one occasion when he balked at the last moment: we were in the

61

bank when he suddenly changed his mind and refused to sign the withdrawal slip, so Vint, with infinite patience, did not press him. Instead, he took him out for a cup of coffee until he had calmed down. They chatted for quite a while about other things—then having regained Dave's confidence, Vinton presented the matter again. This time he was successful and the withdrawal slip was signed, but it took almost a whole afternoon to do this.

I cannot express in words our feelings at having to witness Dave's confusion over handling money matters. Though he was still continuing to improve in other ways, such as driving and getting around by himself, his mind seemed to have lost the ability to see his financial picture in perspective. Knowing how astute he had been formerly made it all the harder to bear. To preserve his self-respect, he still had a checking account in his own name which was used for personal items such as clothes and doctors' or dentists' bills. These checks were usually written under my supervision and signed by him. Quite often he would ask me to write the checks for him.

In other areas of our life I noticed that he was becoming kinder and more gentle toward me; he seemed to sense his need of my help and perhaps not to resent it so much. I am sure that he did feel gratitude for what I had done and recognized to some extent that the things I did were in his best interests. Also, he became quite willing to chat with his neighbors, something he had rarely done in the past. So these were compensations and something to be thankful for. Having had such an encouraging prediction from Dr. Hung, it was much easier for me to be patient with his shortcomings, because I felt certain that he was going to improve to the point where much of the burden of his dependence on me would be removed.

During May of 1977, he improved enough to go for two job interviews. One was for the position of correctional officer in the state juvenile-detention center. The second was with a rehabilitation center which dealt with young people. We knew he had not yet reached the point where he would be able to handle a full-time job, but the fact that he felt able to face an interview was a reason for much rejoicing. What a long way he had come since that January day when the subject of acupuncture was first mentioned. In neither case was there any likelihood that he would be hired, but just the fact of being able to go for an interview did wonders for his self-esteem.

Toward the end of that month, we decided to get another dog. Our little Chihuahua had been put to sleep about a year before, although we still had the English setter. We had tried to adopt a Chihuahua from the pound the winter before, but he had turned out to be very highly strung, nervous, and sometimes for no reason at all would turn vicious. We saw an advertisement in the "nickel ads" of a local classified paper. It was for a Chihuahua-poodle cross, three months old, and the price of twenty dollars included his dog house! It was on Memorial Day when we went over to see him—a pouring wet day. Dave had been excited all morning about another new addition to the family, and it was hard to hold him back from going over to see the dog at eight o'clock in the morning. The family who owned him consisted of a married couple with two little girls, about five and seven years old. They had decided not to keep him as the mother worked full time, which meant that he was left alone in the house all day. When we opened the door, a delightful little black-and-white puppy barked at us, then ran back to protect his two young ladies. We decided at once to take him, and I can remember the mother picked him up and deposited him in my arms. Dave's reactions were slow that day. While I was talking to the owner, he hovered in the background, seeming not to know why he was there. He picked up the dog house, then put it down again, almost forgetting to take it when we left—I had to remind him twice to carry it out to the car for me. Our new puppy stood undecided on the front steps—apparently he had hardly ever been outside the house—and since it was raining hard, it must have seemed a strange and alien world to him. We finally had to lift him off the steps and carry him to the car. He settled in at once, and was a great joy to us and really good therapy for Dave, who spent many hours gloating over him and seeing that he was comfortable. This little dog was destined to be our joy and comfort through four most devastating years. The pleasure he gave to

Dave during hospital visits was touching to see.

To see if Dave could maintain his improvement, the acupuncture treatments had now been reduced to twice a month instead of once a week. At about this time, Dr. Hung suggested that to help him adapt socially, it would be a good idea for Dave to keep a diary. He should enter the events of each day in detail; places he had been, people he had seen, future appointments. This would get him to keep his mind focused as well as reminding him what day of the week it was, and he could refer back to it to get facts established in his memory. This met with mixed success. I had to keep at him constantly to remind him. He would take the diary in to his appointments with Dr. Hung and would be questioned about it. If nothing else, it was good mental exercise, but I noticed that his attention span when he was writing was very short. He would start off well and then after a few words, would trail off and lose his train of thought.

It must have been about the middle of June when I noticed that he was not improving any more, and sometimes seemed to be sliding back to his old ways. Examples of this were going in and out of doors—he was always on the wrong side. He would open a door to go out, then shut it again, staying on the same side. This would be repeated when he got outside and closed the door; he would open and shut it several times before deciding whether to be in or out. His coordination and concentration were not too good when trying to help me around the house or in the garden. He would pick up a spade, do some digging in a spasmodic way, then leave a huge gap and start again in a completely different part of the flower bed. A simple job like cleaning the sink would take him ten or fifteen minutes, and he would do a good job of wiping down parts of a table or the kitchen counter, but then leave big areas untouched. His sense of sequence in completing such jobs appeared to have gone, unless reminded all the time.

I mentioned several of these things to Dr. Hung at our next appointment, and he told me that all acupuncture could do now was to keep him on a plateau. In other words, it had done the maximum that could be expected. Still, I did not feel too discouraged because overall he was so much better than five months before, and I still clung to the hope that our miracle of healing might be a reality. Having got this far, who would want to think otherwise?

The Fourth of July holiday that year was spent with Vinton and Maria. We went on a picnic to Silver Falls State Park and had a really wonderful day together. I felt so thankful for the company and support of these two outstanding friends. They had seen us through so many desperate times during the past year, and had always been unswerving in their loyalty. How priceless are devoted friends such as these. That day, Dave seemed content to go along with whatever was suggested. He basked in the assurance of our goodwill and support, but it was a strange place for him, and at times he was not in touch with what was going on around him. An open-air wedding was going on in one part of the grounds, so he and Vint stopped for a while to join in the festivities. This made a good subject for the diary which he wrote next day. He did all right until he came to a description of what the bride wanted to do . . . but then his memory failed again. I tried to keep him at it, but when under pressure he became petulant and gave up easily.

The doctor questioned him at his next appointment about this day out. Again, he could remember the general outline of the day, but when asked for details he went blank. As a further rehabilitation, Dr. Hung mentioned that some light volunteer work might be helpful, if possible with people who had some of the same symptoms, so that he could feel useful. Accordingly, I contacted an agency that helped senior citizens. Dave had always been good with older people—patient, understanding, and seemingly able to talk to them in a way they could understand and relate to. In the past I had noticed that when talking to someone much older than himself, it had seemed to bring out the best in him.

It was mid-July when we went in for an interview, and I remember that morning I didn't feel too happy about him. He drove the car in and had considerable difficulty parking, almost backing into the car behind him, so I had to yell at him to look out. This put us both on edge and I felt anxious and ill at ease as we walked into the office. While Dave was filling out his application, I had a chance to talk to the director, Mr. Nielsen, alone and explained as clearly as I could about his illness. Dave handled himself well; I was always amazed at the good public front he could present, but he took a long time to complete his application. After that, I left them alone for a while, thinking it would be easier for Mr. Nielsen to make his own evaluation of Dave without me in the background. It was agreed that he would start on a trial basis the following week. The work involved visiting elderly people in their homes or apartments, doing shopping, or taking them to medical and other appointments. Finding out what their needs were and trying to keep them as active and in touch with life as possible. He would be accompanied by a staff member until he got an idea of what was needed, and would work with the same person until he felt comfortable enough to go out on his own.

The following Tuesday morning I drove him down to the agency. We had decided that half a day would be more than enough to begin with, and then he would take the bus home. It seemed that we were on the verge of another beginning, and I felt relieved that he would be doing something to make him feel needed and worthwhile. I hoped and prayed that the stimulation of this work would help him to maintain and build upon the improvement already gained.

When he returned home that afternoon, he was in a silent, pensive mood. He was obviously relieved to be home and made a big fuss over the dogs, but never mentioned how his morning had gone. Naturally, I asked about it and he wasn't too enthusiastic. Coming home on the bus, he hadn't been able to find the right change for his fare and had felt very embarrassed. I was not surprised that he felt this way. He had not worked for more than a year now, and it must have felt like plunging into cold water after so long. I wonder, too, if perhaps he didn't remember much of what he'd done that morning? He would have tried to make a good impression, and the effort of trying to keep this up may have made his recollection even more blurred for the time being. However, I was encouraged by the fact that they had asked him to go in again the next day, but also somewhat surprised, as I had told Mr. Nielsen that he would need to take it easy to start with. He didn't seem unduly fatigued, and after his second day of work came home much more interested and with some constructive suggestions as to how some aspects of the job might be handled better, so I urged him to talk about this to the volunteer who was training him.

Once more, they had asked him to go in for the third day in succession. That morning, when he woke up he said, "I don't want to go in today." If I had really listened to him, I would have known he was telling me that he had had enough for that week, and I would have had the wisdom to let it rest there, to call the agency and say that those two mornings had been sufficient. But no, I persisted that he go in; I felt that perhaps he needed to be pushed at this point to overcome his own natural reluctance. I tried to encourage him by saying that they appreciated his work and his willingness to try. He took a long time to bathe, shave, and get dressed, but eventually took off in his car. Part of my reason for wanting him to go was that he had been without a purpose for so long that surely any outlet such as this must be constructive; also to be truthful there were times when it was a relief to have him out of the house. So once again, I made a decision I was to regret. My own day was busy and fulfilling; I was able to catch up on a lot of things without interruption, and it felt good to have the house to myself for a while.

I had expected him home soon after lunch, but mid-afternoon came and he had not returned. I was not too worried. Perhaps he had gone to the Elks Club after work. He had been a member for several years and in the past had enjoyed playing racquetball there, so he could have dropped in to renew some old friendships.

When it was almost five o'clock and he had not appeared, I called the agency. No, he had not been in at all today—they had expected him and had tried to reach him at home but there was no answer. I felt a sense of panic deep within me; it was a struggle to keep my head at that moment and not be overwhelmed by the

67

possibilities of what might have happened. The next three hours were a time of immense desolation and gnawing anxiety. How was I to handle this? Should I go out and try to look for him . . . but where would I begin? How much longer should I wait? When do I report him missing? By 8:00 P.M. I had still heard nothing and kept hoping that the phone would ring saying he was on his way home. I had to turn to someone for help, for reassurance, to someone who cared and would be willing to listen. I called Mary Ellen Cowen, a good friend in my prayer group and told her the whole story. After listening compassionately, she asked if I needed someone to come over and be with me. I said no, but would she please pray for his safety and that he would return unharmed.

It must have been entirely due to her prayers that I was able to sleep that night. I hadn't expected to, but I sensed that I was not allowed to feel the full extent of this horror. In the chapter on Acceptance I have described how at times a protective veil was thrown around my feelings, and this was exactly what happened that night, releasing me from my worst fears for the time being.

The next morning I was due to go in to William Temple House for a day of counseling. Somehow I managed to get through the morning, but the pressure of this nightmare was building inside me, and after lunch I told Father Abbott what had happened and that I must go home. I had telephoned the house several times but there had been no answer. I arrived home about 2:15. Oh, what joy and relief it was to see his car parked in front of the garage. It was parked all crooked to be sure, but still in one piece and intact.

I felt limp with apprehension as I went into the house, not knowing how I would find him. The bedroom curtains were drawn and he was lying on the bed in a dazed state, exhausted and unable to make sense. His speech was incoherent, most of the sentences not hanging together or in any logical sequence. About all I could get out of him was: "There were bright lights and the traffic was going 'round and 'round. I was in the car and it was very cold." He must have spent most of the night in the car, perhaps walking around at times trying to get his bearings. He

68

couldn't tell me where he'd been. It was a miracle that he'd been able to find his way home after more than twenty-four hours, undoubtedly lost most of the night and not knowing what to do to help himself.

One of the worst things about this disease is that there is so much I'll never know because he was incapable of telling me. I do know, however, without a doubt, that he was protected during those lonely hours, and to those who say there is no God who watches over us, what better proof could there be than his safe return?

I made him as comfortable as I could, gave him a light meal, and then knew I must telephone the doctor. In a house as small as ours it was impossible to talk privately and the last thing he needed now was to hear me discussing his condition, so I went over to Gwen's house, where I poured out my distress. We had had so much hope these past three months, but now it was dwindling again. My sudden arrival surprised Gwen, but without asking any questions, she knew I was in desperate need. I telephoned Dr. Hung, describing in detail all that had taken place. This was definitely a regression, he said, evidently brought on by the pressure of the volunteer work which had been too much. Our intentions had been so good, but who was to know how much he was capable of at this stage? Appearances were deceptive, as on the surface he had seemed so much better than was actually the case. My mistake had been to push him into more than he could handle. It was a costly mistake and brought on a regression that might have been delayed for sometime, but which eventually would have happened because of the relentless nature of the disease. The doctor told me not to be too discouraged, but to bring him back in for a treatment the following Tuesday. He would try once more to stabilize him as much as was possible under the circumstances.

The next few days were a kind of limbo . . . after a good night's rest, he recovered to the point that he made sense again, but didn't have much energy and couldn't remember anything about those lost hours. His appetite began to change and he ate very little and had no enthusiasm for foods he had once enjoyed. Again, he spent a lot of time sorting out his desk, going through

69

old letters and papers, some of which he would throw away, and some he would take into the bedroom and put away in different places. This constant moving of papers caused extreme frustration to me, as I was trying to keep bills, accounts, and legal documents in order. Invariably he would go through them and misplace them, not meaning to, but he had simply lost his grasp of organization.

Shortly after this setback, he again became more childlike and affectionate toward me and tried so hard to be helpful. It seemed as though more of his defenses were gone since this last episode, and instead of fighting against his dependence on me, he was gradually accepting it. Thus July ended. After his acupuncture treatment the last week of that month, we decided not to continue as they had achieved the maximum that could be expected. In no way do I regret this course. It gave him three extra months of much better quality life which he otherwise would not have had. True, our hopes were raised to a point where we expected the improvement might be maintained for quite a long time. Always in the background was that desire for a miracle of healing; I had counted so much on that when he began to improve, but it was not to be. So once again our hopes were dashed—once more we had to accept the fact that the damage to his brain was extensive and irreversible. The symptoms had been lessened, but underneath the outward improvement, its progress continued irrevocably.

5. Regression

"Out of the depths have I called to thee, O Lord"

The first week of August, 1977 was very hot. I had been fortunate enough to be able to get away to the beach for a few days
soon after Dave's setback, which helped enormously in building
up my strength again to face the next phase of our life. This
brief respite had been like an oasis in a parched desert. While
I was gone, Vinton and Delores had kept an eye on Dave for
me. He did not have much ambition to go out of the house at
this time, but would occasionally drive short distances to get himself a meal. Vinton took him out for a day, and another neighbor,
Mr. Johnston, came over and visited two or three times. I had
left my telephone number down at the beach with Vinton, so he
could let me know if there was any urgent need.

About two days after my return, Dave seemed a lot better—
perhaps the time apart had helped us both. It was a Thursday,
I remember, and I had an appointment that afternoon to see
Vinton alone to talk over some matters concerning the conservatorship, and the implications of Dave's recent severe lapse. Vinton, as usual more perceptive than I, had noticed that he was
slipping before I did, and it was helpful to get his views even
though I dreaded the downhill road which was now so clearly
before us.

That same afteroon, Dave said he was going to drive in
to the Elks Club for a while. I knew this was a risk, but he seemed
to want to get out of the house, and at least I knew where he was

71

going. He left and about ten minutes later drove in again. This happened twice, and I really don't know the reason except that he may have forgotten where he was supposed to be going. The third time he left and didn't come back so I assumed he had made it down to the club all right.

I arrived home about 4:30 P.M., but Dave was still out. I started to prepare dinner, and then thought it would be a good idea to call the Elks Club to see if he had in fact been there. They said he was not in the Club at that moment, but had been seen there earlier in the afternoon. This time, I knew what to do. I got in my car and drove straight down to the Club. Dave's car was parked outside the front entrance, and he was sitting in it, just staring into space. He didn't seem surprised to see me, and smiled as though he had expected me. He got out of the car when he saw me and I asked him if he was ready to go home. He was not unduly upset or out of touch this time, but totally incapable of knowing what to do, why he was down there, or what was the next step. If I hadn't appeared on the scene, most likely he would have been gone again all night, with perhaps disastrous results. I knew he couldn't possibly drive himself home, so we went into the club together to ask if he might park his car in their garage overnight. I explained that he was not well and unable to drive at the moment, and told them I would pick up his car the following morning. I noticed that while we were in the club, he was sort of disoriented, looking about him as though these were unfamiliar surroundings when in fact he had been there many times. He was most gracious in thanking the receptionist for her help, and there was a gentleness and vulnerability about him that was surprising considering his inability to help himself. One would expect him to be defensive, upset, and agitated, but this was not so. I have wondered since what it was that drew him back to the club. Did he still have happy memories of times spent there? Of racquetball games and his friendship with the sports manager, Tye? It must have represented a place where he felt secure and accepted, even if specific memories of people he had known had faded.

I was thankful to get him home before a repeat of the previous disaster. I dread to think what might have happened if he had been lost and wandering for another twenty-four hours. Earlier, I spoke about the heat making the symptoms much worse, and I wonder if that is what happened, because on each occasion, a burning August sun was beating down on the car, and this could have caused him to succumb more quickly to confusion and disorientation. It would be interesting to me to know whether others with this disease have had the same experience when exposed to hot sun.

The following day, Vinton and Maria invited us to go down and have dinner with them. Once more, it was hot and Dave was sitting on the sunny side of the car. When we left, he was in a cheerful mood, seemingly without any aftereffects of his outing the day before. He was chatty to begin with and we had good conversation for about the first half of the drive. Then gradually, he became silent, and the next time I spoke to him, hardly bothered to reply. He was shifting uncomfortably in his seat and it was clear that something was wrong. Since I knew it was hot on his side, I opened both front and back windows and told him to do the same. Shortly after this, he lurched forward in his seat, holding his head, and shouted, "I am out of it, I am out of it." I didn't know what to do, and a cold feeling of panic gripped me. I tried to get him to tell me what was wrong, where he was hurting. He couldn't answer except to writhe and obviously didn't know what was happening to him. I slowed down and tried to comfort him, telling him we'd soon be there. A bit later on, we were driving through heavy traffic in Salem, and a car drew up alongside with its radio blaring. Dave grabbed my arm, shouting, "We have to stop, Claire, he told us to halt."

He seemed convinced we were being followed by the police and his interpretation of the radio noise was evidently to him their instructions. With profound relief, I realized we only had about three more miles to go, but he was uneasy, restless, and out of touch until we got to their house. I have never been more thankful to come to the end of a drive than on that day. There was a feeling of intense fear and also unreality; again these happenings as I lived through them had a dream-like quality—like a nightmare that will vanish as soon as one wakes up. It couldn't really be happening to Dave in this way; why hadn't the doctors told me to expect this kind of thing? Once inside the house, he relaxed and was able to enter fairly well into our evening together. I did notice, though, that whenever he looked out of the window, he was "seeing things," hallucinating, and there was a fearful expression on his face. Vinton noticed it too, and drew the curtains.

All through dinner, I was trying to sort out the turmoil within me. I badly needed a moment alone with either Vint or Maria to tell them what had happened, and was able to do this when they were both outside in the garden for a few minutes. Up until now, I had never had to face the stark terror of seeing him go through a seizure like this. A grim, desolate wasteland had come into our lives, and I had to realize that there might well be more episodes like this in the future. Undoubtedly, the most terrifying aspect of Alzheimer's Disease is its unpredictability; one cannot be prepared for the next stage because its totally uncertain just what that next stage will be.

The heat wave continued, and Sunday, August 7, dawned clear and still, with the promise of yet another sweltering day. I went to church that morning, and Dave stayed at home. He seemed peaceful and it was surprising to me that after these dreadful episodes, he would return the next day to an almost normal state. After lunch, he asked me if I would go up and pay a bill for him at the racquet club where he was a member. He seemed quite normal and at peace when I left; we sat down and talked for a few minutes, and I remember being encouraged by the fact that he knew the bill should be paid, without getting resentful or hostile.

I was gone for about an hour, and when I came back, he was sitting at the dining room table in the same place as when I left. There was a ghastly stiffness and rigidity about him. He was staring blankly into space and didn't even seem to notice I was back. I spoke to him, trying to get some response, but he seemed to be transfixed and unable to do anything except stare and stare blankly, as if in another world altogether. I asked him

74

if he would like to move to the sofa where he would be more comfortable, but he seemed terrified even to try moving to another part of the room. I forced myself to act as normally as possible and decided it was no good trying to make him do anything until this phase (whatever it was) had passed.

We had a little guest cottage separate from the house, so I went over there to try and calm myself enough to deal with this totally new and unexpected crisis. I prayed in desperation for guidance and courage. My feelings were churning within—horror, grief, fear, dread; what to do, where to turn. *What does this mean? Will I have to face many more times like these, and if so, how can I ever find the strength to face them? What can I do to help him?* Oh God, help me, I feel so hopeless, so lost. As if in answer, the first lines of a verse came to me:

> Take my grief and let it be
> Consecrated, Lord to thee
> Take my anguish and despair
> Make of them a heartfelt prayer
> Grant us, Lord, thy inner peace
> From all doubt and pain release.
> Thou art closer than we know
> Ready to supply our need
> Help us, Lord, in times distraught
> To know that thou art there to lead
> Grace and mercy, love unfailing
> Knowledge, peace and wisdom flow
> From thine infinite abundance
> To all who suffer here below.
> Teach us, Lord, to lean on thee
> To trust the still, small voice within
> All things unto thee committed
> Eternal joy and blessing bring.

For He has promised, "I will never fail you nor forsake you."
This was written in the space of about an hour on that grim Sunday afternoon when the bottom seemed to have dropped out

75

of our lives. That is, the life we had led together for thirteen years was now drastically changing in a way over which we had no control whatsoever. I know that this poem was given to me as a comfort and an assurance that I was not alone. There was one who cared and understood. There is no way I could possibly have written this by myself, or out of my own inspiration. I was much too emotionally drained and horror-struck to have written anything coherent at that moment. Yet, as I was given these words, I felt my strength returning and that there was meaning, even in this dreadful afternoon. It was a sign we were not forsaken. While this was being written, I had to concentrate and in so doing had to forget for the time being Dave's ghastly dilemma. So in a way it was therapy too—to force my mind away from something impossible to deal with all at once. I was going to need strength for the rest of that day, because things weren't going to get better. All that afternoon he sat in the same chair, scarcely moving, occasionally turning his head slightly, but always with the same expression, a trancelike, fixed stare. I tried to do a few chores in the garden and around the house, thinking that perhaps my moving in and out would break his trance. It seemed to be an effort for him to say anything and he couldn't gather his thoughts together in a logical way. Mostly, he would just answer in a monosyllable, with his mind apparently paralyzed and unable to focus. On one of my journeys from the cabin to the house a voice within me said, "He's dying isn't he?" It was in the form of a question, and yet it was a statement of fact at the same time, and immediately I denied it: "Oh, no, it couldn't be true—it's much too cruel to contemplate." But I knew unmistakably that the question was right and the answer was yes, however much I might deny it.

At dinner time, Dave hardly ate anything and his movements were stiff and awkward. Once or twice, he half-rose from his chair, as though to move away, but then sat down again, seemingly too frightened to venture anywhere else. I think he was only half-aware of my comings and goings, but I still kept moving, thinking that eventually it might help him to snap out of it.

At about ten o'clock, I got ready for bed, now thoroughly

worn out, and suggested that he should do the same. It took quite awhile, but finally he came to the bedroom door, pushed it open, and stared into the room as though it was completely unfamiliar. Then he got down on his knees and looked underneath the bed. I couldn't believe what I was seeing. He moved stiffly, like a sleepwalker, to the edge of the bed and sat down, still fully dressed. He made no attempt to undress, but just remained there, as rigid as before. I couldn't get him to lie down and he didn't seem sleepy at all, just rigid and tense. It was impossible to sleep with him sitting on the edge of the bed, so eventually I went out and lay down on the sofa. I don't know how much longer he sat there gazing into space; I left the bedroom door open and from time to time would look in to see if he had lain down, but it was well past midnight when I finally dropped off into a fitful sleep, and at that time he was still sitting upright in the same place. It had now been more than twelve hours since this had happened and I had no idea how long it might go on.

Somehow, the night passed and I suppose it must have been about four o'clock the next morning when I tiptoed into the bedroom and found with immense relief that he was lying down, asleep. He had not undressed, but had pulled the bedspread up over him. He awoke at about eight, and seemed much better; was not rigid or speechless anymore, although his movements were rather slow and deliberate. While he was shaving, I called Vinton to tell him what had happened, and he said he would come up in about an hour to talk the whole thing over and discuss what the next step should be. He must have had no difficulty at all in sensing the desperation in my voice. When he arrived, Dave indicated that he would like to talk to him alone, so I respected this wish and left them together for about an hour.

Vinton later told me that Dave wanted to tell him about the people who were patrolling the house and grounds; he had seen "them" driving up and down the street checking on the house, and felt sure he was under surveillance. Also there was a strange light on in the bedroom, and he didn't feel it was safe to go in there. That wherever he went, he was being watched. Vinton did his best to dispel these fears, but to Dave they were very real.

When I got back things were more peaceful, at least for the time being.

It was decided that we should see another neurologist for advice as to how to handle these present circumstances. Accordingly, an appointment was made with Dr. Harold Sanger for Thursday, August 11. The two days in between were quiet and uneventful with, thankfully, no repeat of Sunday's dreadful episode. Dave did not seem to resent this appointment with a new doctor; he was quite open to being taken and evidently now accepted the fact that we were doing all we could to help him. When we left the house, I noticed that he was uncomfortable outside; he was all right once inside the car, but seemed fearful and insecure when out in the open.

The doctor gave him a very thorough examination. Before he saw Dave I talked to him alone to bring him up to date on the latest events. During his examination he gave Dave three words to remember: Red, table, dog, and said later on he would ask him to recall those words. He was direct, very experienced, and somewhat austere, but gave me a feeling that he knew his job thoroughly and was conscientious. On the whole, Dave responded quite well to his questions, but became confused when asked to look at a certain point on the wall when his eyes were being examined. He didn't comprehend at all, and looked everywhere but at that point. Also, I noticed that he had no reflexes when tapped on the knee and the back of his heel. When he was dressed, we went back into the doctor's office and he gave us some clear directions. Keep him busy, not only mentally, but with his hands; get him to read if possible. Give him IQ tests, mathematical tests; take up sketching, drawing, or any hobby that would require concentration. At one point, he said bluntly, "You are not to sit and stare." Then he asked Dave to remember what the three words were he was to remember. "Red, table . . ." a long pause, and he couldn't remember the third one. Overall, the doctor seemed to think he was doing better than a lot of patients at a similar stage in the disease. At this first appointment, he had not seen pictures of the brain scan, but sent for them, and told us to come back again four weeks later.

As we left the clinic and walked out into the parking lot, Dave stared around him, and once again seemed to be seeing things. I opened the car door, but he wouldn't get in, staring up and down the street. He said, "I am sure they're going to nail us this time." It was quite a few minutes later before I could break through and get him into the car.

That weekend, we followed up on the doctor's advice and went out together to buy some drawing and sketching pads with instruction books on how to start. Dave had been impressed by Dr. Sanger, who had not talked down to him but had treated him "man to man." "I feel I could be really helped by some therapy from him," he said. During the next couple of weeks, we settled down to our sketching and drawing, general knowledge tests and math tests.

Dave was quite willing to try, and if I sat down with him, he would stay at his drawing for quite a long time, but needed my encouragement and support. Also he had little or no initiative of his own by this time. On general knowledge tests he was best at remembering past presidents of the U.S., and quite a few of the political questions he would answer accurately. He did quite well on geographical questions concerning the capitals of other countries. One day, I tried to get him to play checkers again, a game he had always enjoyed, but after a couple of moves he just couldn't remember the object of the game or what he was supposed to do. On simple mathematical problems he did quite well, but when it came to subtraction he had difficulty. He would write out the figures and try to use the method he had learned of subtracting when in school, but often he couldn't complete the problem, would get half the answer and then lose track. When he tried to concentrate extra hard, it seemed that the block was worse. One day he said, "Claire, it's as though a wall goes up when I try to remember what to do." At times like these, I didn't know what to say. I just tried to be as encouraging as possible and when he was able to do a problem well, I gave him abundant praise. In arithmetic, I noticed, he was not consistent; some days he could subtract quite well, but the next time, he couldn't recall the mechanics of what he had done previously.

79

At about this time, he went through a phase of being afraid to leave the house and would ask before we left if we had permission to go out—was it safe? One Sunday afternoon, we were sitting at the dining room table working on drawing and sketching when the telephone rang. It was Vinton, saying that he had his son Fred and daughter-in-law staying, and would we like to meet them for dinner. Thinking that Dave would be more than happy to go, I told him the news. To my amazement, he said, "Claire, I don't think we should go—I don't think it's safe to leave." Try as I would, I couldn't convince him otherwise. I felt bitterly disappointed, as an evening out would have made a most welcome break in our routine. I explained how he felt to Vinton, so instead he said they would drop by for a short visit. Even then Dave was too frightened to go outside the front door to greet them. He stood hesitantly just inside and showed relief when they finally left and the door could be safely closed again. He genuinely felt this way; I could see by his expression that the fear was real, so there was nothing for it but to cancel this outing.

Quite often after this episode, when we were alone together in the house, he would look around the room with a dazed expression and say, "This isn't our house, is it?" Or, "Is it safe to go into the bedroom—are we alone here?" Gradually, I suppose, his recognition of familiar surroundings was dwindling. When this happened, I would gently remind him that he was indeed at home and that all was well.

Ruth and Nolan, having heard about his setbacks, contacted us and planned to come up and stay for about a week over the Labor Day weekend, and their visit was a real blessing to both of us. Nolan, who is extremely capable with his hands, worked with Dave putting together a model ship and an airplane. I shall always be grateful for the cheerful, spontaneous way he spent hours keeping Dave occupied and stimulated. Even though his contribution to the building of these two models was small, it gave him such pleasure to be included in the project, and Nolan would consult him all the time about what they should do next. He then got a "do-it-yourself" painting kit and got Dave involved in painting a picture of an English setter, again asking his advice all the time, making him feel he was important and that his opinion was needed. What better therapy could there have been? This also gave me some free time to get away with Ruth, without feeling that Dave was alone in the house; in addition it removed the burden of being his constant supervisor all the time.

One Sunday morning after we came home from church, we decided it would be fun to go out for lunch for a change. It had been about three weeks since Dave's refusal to go out for a meal, so I hoped that by this time he would have got over his fear, especially since he enjoyed Ruth and Nolan's company so much and would feel secure going out with them. He really didn't want to go, but we finally persuaded him and it didn't work out too well. He had difficulty deciding what to eat and looked fearfully around the restaurant. He was obviously relieved when the time came to pay the bill and leave. In fact, he handed me his wallet and told me to pay our share, which was surprising and totally opposite to his usual defense against my involvement with his money.

During that week, the time had come again for us to go back and see Dr. Sanger. It had been a month since our last visit. When reminded about the appointment, Dave resisted. I am sure he didn't want to go back because it confirmed to him that he was seriously ill, and who wants to be reminded of a hopeless situation? So I really couldn't blame him. I decided to go alone, and it gave me the opportunity to ask the doctor some specific questions about what to expect. I asked if this condition might lead to a stroke, but he said that usually this was not so, but he would gradually lose control of all his functions and there might be seizures. Eventually, he would have to be taken care of in a nursing home or some other kind of institution. It would be a matter of long-term care which would, of course, be very expensive. Therefore, I should try and manage at home for as long as I possibly could and get some help to relieve me. By this time he had received copies of the EMI scan taken in July of 1976, and told me that in his opinion Dave had what he called a "moderately severe dementia" with extensive damage to the cerebral cortex. The symptoms would get worse. When I pressed him for details as to just how much worse, he didn't answer but looked down at his hands. This gesture told me more than any words could have done.

In thinking about the reasons why doctors are so evasive when pressed for answers about the progress of this disease, I believe they feel unable to predict with any accuracy just what course it is going to take, or how long. It seems that each case is different depending upon what parts of the brain are affected. Normally the progress is very slow, as in Dave's case, but some go very fast. Since there is no known cure and nothing that can arrest it, they feel helpless and frustrated. Scientifically, I am sure a doctor wants to give as accurate a prediction as possible, but in the case of Alzheimer's, this cannot be done. Therefore, many of the answers they give to questions such as I asked have to be speculation, and in some cases they may have been sued for giving information that did not turn out to be right. Then, it must be extremely painful and difficult to pass on this hopeless diagnosis in a way that can be accepted by the patient and his family. Also, a doctor must weigh just how much he should tell. How much can the family bear at this point? Does he know them well enough to tell the whole truth, or is he in fact doing them a service by not telling everything he knows? It may be quite enough for them to handle each stage as it comes. And so, from experience, I think I can understand a doctor's point of view. He may well be trying to save the family unnecessary grief knowing full well that when each change occurs, then it will be time enough to face that stage of deterioration and live through it step by step.

In the beginning, I felt it was my right to know everything about each stage so that I could be prepared, and yet the anticipated dread of what may happen can be even more devastating. Are we ever really prepared for the major crises of our lives? So, in a very real sense I see now that their reluctance in telling me all the details had a reason, and perhaps from a professional point of view, it is the best way to handle a terminal disease of this kind.

One afternoon, I came home from my volunteer work and found Dave sitting at the dining-room table with an overturned glass of milk in his hand. Once more, he was in that now all-too-familiar rigid pose, staring ahead, while the dogs sat close by, lapping up the milk which had trickled down the side of his chair on to the floor. This time my return brought him back to reality. I disguised my shock at finding him in this condition, cleared up the mess, and then started to get dinner ready. That evening, he seemed frightened and would hardly let me out of his sight. From time to time, muscle spasms would run down his left shoulder and arm, and he would shake and quiver, looking 'round the room with a terrified expression. I stayed close to him all that evening, not knowing what to expect, and trying to reassure him. I suppose this was a form of mild seizure, and at about that time, I cut my volunteer work to two half-days a week, realizing that soon it might no longer be safe to leave him at home alone.

I also started inquiries as to some kind of help to give me relief at home. I called my local county nursing association and a home-health agency, but neither of them were very helpful. He was not a nursing case; the kind of services they gave involved bathing, changing dressings, house cleaning, cooking, help with getting dressed, or physical therapy, none of which he needed at this time. What he did need was someone to keep him occupied mentally and be a companion, but this need was not being met by either of these agencies. There was a sense of deep disappointment as I finally realized there was no agency that covered the kind of help I wanted. It was a low time for us after Ruth and Nolan left. It had been so much help having them there, and Dave said one morning, "You know, I really miss Nolan," and I am sure he did. I wished so much that they lived closer. However, there was a bright spot in that September. I got tickets for a musical *The Tales of Hoffman,* and since Dave was now beginning to overcome his fear of going outside the house, this would really be something to look forward to. I was thankful that he was willing to go and indeed seemed eager for an evening out. Our seats were in the first balcony, and we arrived about fifteen minutes early. He began to be restless, evidently forgetting why we were there, and I had visions of having to leave even before the curtain went up. However, all was well, and he seemed to thoroughly enjoy the music, the drama, the color, and pageantry.

During the intermission, I had to take him to the men's room, and there were some anxious moments waiting for him to come out; he took a long time, and I am sure if I had not waited for him, he wouldn't have been able to find his way back to his seat.

The second act was quite long, and I noticed that he was getting restless toward the end of it, so I asked him if he would like to leave. He said yes, and so we left during the interval between the second and third acts, walking out arm in arm to the car. I felt it was a triumph that we had been able to have this happy evening together; it stands out as a lovely memory during those last months when he was at home. Anything that brings joy at a time like this is something to be treasured.

Later on that week we had an appointment with the dentist. It was a yearly checkup for Dave and I drove him in. I asked the receptionist how long it was likely to be and she told me about forty-five minutes. I didn't think it was necessary to tell her about his condition, but just said I'd be back to pick him up and then went off to do some shopping. When I arrived back at the dentist's office they told me he had left a few minutes before. I had never dreamt that he wouldn't wait for me, and with a sinking heart, I left and began to look for him. However, he was in familiar territory and probably would not be far away, so I decided to walk a few blocks, feeling sure I would soon find him.

With growing anxiety I searched each street up and down for a distance of about half a mile. I was getting hot and frustrated—how could it be so difficult to find him in a small town? I went back and got the car and drove around the whole area, covering the places where I thought he would be most likely to go, including the Elks Club. I went in there and told them to be on the lookout for him. Inevitably I had to tell them part of his problem, and that he sometimes became disoriented. By this time, at least an hour had passed since he had walked out of the dentist's office. Perhaps he had taken a bus home or had started to walk that way, as we were only three miles from the center of town, so I drove slowly home fully expecting to see him walking somewhere along that familiar road.

I arrived at the house and walked in to find it quiet and empty. The dogs were outside in our fenced yard, enjoying a sunny, late September afternoon. Once inside, I took stock of what was happening and how I was going to deal with it. I remember going into the bedroom and throwing the window wide open. I stood for a few moments looking out on that garden—its rhododendrons, azaleas, roses, and trees—a garden I had loved and tended and which had come to mean so much to me during our thirteen years of marriage. I had expected to feel panic, but instead a deep feeling of serenity came to me—I must accept what had just happened as normal; it was a reality of life now and not something to be surprised about. It seemed to sweep away all questions as to where he might be and give me a release; the burden was not mine alone. I then telephoned Gwen and shared the whole experience with her, including my new-found feeling of peace. She said she would drive in and take a look for him. I also called the dentist's office and told them the whole story and to be sure and let me know if by chance he did come back. They were really concerned and told me to let them know as soon as I had found him.

The last resort and the one I dreaded most was calling the police, but there seemed to be no other alternative. Always, explaining Dave's condition was a painful business, but it had to be done. I gave a full description of his appearance and what he was wearing. About half an hour later they called back to say they had found him; he was standing outside the real estate office where he had once worked, apparently lost and not making any attempt to help himself. With a sense of overwhelming relief, I begged them to stay with him till I could get there, but they said that was impossible because they already had two other emergencies that afternoon and not enough personnel to cover them. I drove back in as fast as I dared, and mercifully he was still standing in exactly the same place. I parked behind the building, immune to the curious stares of those inside who had been watching him for some time. All I could feel was gratitude that he was safe and sound. He must have felt hot and thirsty standing there for so long, as it had developed into a really hot afternoon.

I wonder so much how far he had walked in the two or three hours that he was missing, but as usual, he was not able to tell me. He didn't seem upset or agitated about what had happened; it was as though his sense of reality was blurred and the fact that he had been missing again didn't register.

I gave him lunch when we got home, and he ate with a good appetite. Then he relaxed for the rest of the afternoon. Since leaving the office, he had been on his feet for close to three hours and heaven only knows what mileage he had covered.

Toward the end of September he appeared to stabilize again, and didn't seem to get any worse. This lasted for about two months, and there were no more seizures, so far as I know. He became increasingly helpful and more loving toward me; of course he was much more dependent on me now, and it was out of the question for him to drive. He would try to help me with housework, vacuuming, and also in the garden. His intentions were so good, but often he was little or no help. He would plug in the vacuum for me and I would start to clean; long before I was finished he would pull the cord out of the plug thinking it was all done. Then he would plug it back in again, and the whole procedure would be repeated. If it hadn't been for our tragedy, this might have been comic, but as it was, often I didn't know whether to laugh or cry or scream. I was on the verge of hysteria many times during those final months when he was still at home. He was quite unaware of his mixed-up reactions and one day when I broke down and cried because of frustration over his sincere, yet bumbling efforts to help, he was so kind and understanding. "We've got to help each other, Claire," he said. I couldn't possibly be angry, but these kind of everyday irritations took their toll.

There was so little he could do now because his attention span was almost nil, and like a child he would soon lose interest in what he was doing and drift off to something else. If not helping, he would follow me around the house, hovering over me and unwilling to let me out of his sight. To get away sometimes, I would try to slip out without him noticing. If I took him shopping with me, I had to watch constantly in case he walked away and got lost, so it was easier to go alone. But the guilt I often felt at leaving him was also overwhelming, so I would not stay out long. If I had planned to be out for the afternoon, I would try to do something with him in the morning, either take him for a drive or walk, and before I left I would get him started on some sketching or drawing. He seldom watched TV now, and even when he did, I doubt if he retained much of what he saw. Increasingly, I had an uneasy feeling when I was away from the house for three hours or more, and still I kept trying to find someone who could come in and help.

One day, I braced myself and decided I must face the fact that I would have to start looking at nursing homes; the time was going to come when I could no longer manage at home alone. Gwen went with me the first time. It seemed so unreal—was it really me who was doing this? How would Dave ever accept it? How could I present it to him? The nursing-home administrator was gracious and patient in answering my questions. She showed us around the place, which was one of the more expensive in our area. It was undoubtedly well run and clean. Dave would have to be willing to come in of his own accord without being forced. If he was not willing, he would have to be legally certified. She advised me that I tell him the truth and not make up any stories just to make it easier for myself. The longer we stayed and the more patients we saw, the more depressed I became. Dave was not anywhere near as far gone as most of these. How could I be thinking about putting him in such a place? It was like another bad dream and hope is so strong that even then, I pushed away this hideous prospect. Gwen told me to keep him at home as long as I possibly could, so that I would have no regrets later.

October 1977 was a beautiful month. The autumn colors were vivid and the leaves lingered on the trees well into November, giving a brilliant display of orange, gold, brown, and russet hues. It was during this month that I finally asked Gwen if she would be willing to come in one morning a week and help me out. I would pay her an hourly rate, and it would give me a chance to get out for a while without feeling I had abandoned Dave. We agreed that she would come in Wednesday mornings for about three hours. It was wonderful to have this definite arrangement, and to know that I could safely plan to be away at that time. We had invested in a tape recorder and got some tapes of good choral and orchestral music which he enjoyed and which seemed to have a soothing effect. Sometimes, he would join in when a well-known tune was being sung.

Ruth and Nolan came again for a brief visit, and as always, it was good to see them. Ruth and I went down to Salem one afternoon, leaving Nolan and Dave together working on various things, including a jigsaw puzzle. The evening after they left, we went out for dinner and I could hardly believe how normal Dave seemed that night. He was not confused at all, found his own way to the men's room, and when the bill came, paid it himself without any help from me. These days would again raise hope that perhaps things were not as bad as we thought.

Gwen told me that when she came in Wednesday mornings, she would try and keep Dave occupied in various ways. One day she made cookies and asked him to help her. He was quite interested getting the first batch ready and helped put the mixture on the baking sheet, but when it came to the second batch, he had lost interest. He often talked about his childhood, his days as a Boy Scout and the badges he had earned. He spoke with great affection about his parents—his father's hobbies and the lovely photographs he took of birds and flowers. Gwen asked him if he would have been interested in photography, but he said no, he didn't think it was for him. He almost never talked about the present or future, and never mentioned that he might get better. Sometimes she would take him out for a drive and he enjoyed going to Farrell's for an ice-cream sundae. One day while at Farrell's a birthday party was in progress, and he chatted to all the children and their parents. He seemed to have lost many of his inhibitions and defenses because previously he had always been withdrawn and antisocial except with people he knew well.

Just before Christmas, Gwen took him over to her house and got him busy helping to make candles. He worked quite well until his attention gave out, then he became restless, and kept asking her when I was going to come and pick him up. Once I came in, he would settle down again.

Sometimes they talked about the Bible, and about his mother. He knew she had had tremendous faith and remembered the times as a boy when he used to go to church with her. Gwen asked him if he knew his mother was now in heaven? He said yes, he knew, and that he had seen her in person, which confirmed the vision that he told me about in September, '75 when she appeared to him one night while he was sleeping in her bedroom. I was amazed that he still remembered this; it must have made a deep impression. They talked about what heaven might be like, and Gwen asked what he thought. He said, "I think it will be like a park—perhaps like some of the places I used to go camping when I was a Scout." He apparently never talked about his time in the Marine Corps. It was clear that he had a deep love and loyalty to his mom and dad, and that their example had meant a great deal to him. I think that when they died, he in a sense died, too. His life was too much linked to theirs after he grew up, and since he couldn't seem to find his own stability, he lived on theirs.

The first weekend in November, Vinton kindly took Dave away with him for a weekend so that I could get some rest. They went north up to Tacoma and Seattle, and spent almost a day going over the battleship *Mighty Mo* in Bremerton harbor. Vinton told me Dave obviously enjoyed the trip, but in the motel became very disorganized when taking a bath and dressing. He did some hallucinating while they were driving, but nothing too violent. The two days alone were certainly appreciated—any break at that time was welcome, as the daily grind of both supervising and trying to keep him occupied took a heavy emotional toll.

It became more and more evident how much his memory was deteriorating; an example of this was one day when he said he had something important to tell me. It was a superb autumn day, so we went out into the garden and sat for a while. I asked him what was on his mind, but he couldn't recall it. I could tell by his expression that there was something weighing heavily, but he was not able to express it. He started a sentence two or three times, but then lost the thread of what he wanted to say. Sometimes when this happened, I developed almost a sixth sense of where his thoughts might be, and was able to tune him in.

More frequently now he would have hallucinations. Once he looked out of the living room window and described something he saw hanging in a tree, which was totally beyond my imagination. It sounded like a mixture of a spider's web and an ultramodern painting—a mixed-up jumble of color and design which to him must have been real. Another day, when driving to Salem, he had been gazing out of the window for some time and asked me if I had noticed that there was a hand up there in the sky. He saw bright red on the brass doorknob of our bedroom door, and told me if I couldn't see it too, I must be stupid. What was wrong with me? "Don't try to tell me I am a jerk," he said. I finally decided that it was best to go along with his hallucinations and ask him to describe them fully to me. If I denied them, it made him look even farther out of touch.

Sometimes during this phase, there were embarrassing moments when we went shopping together. On one occasion, we had taken our tape recorder in for repair, and had called at the shop to pick it up. While we were waiting, Dave went behind the counter, walked up to one of the salesmen, and greeted him like a long-lost friend. He did the same thing in a hardware store, and, in thinking about the possible reasons for his doing this, I can only speculate that perhaps unfamiliar faces now appeared familiar to him, or possibly had some connection with his early childhood.

His inner time clock started to go awry, and he had no sense of when it was time to go to bed or of mealtimes. At bedtime, when I reminded him, he would start to undress, then promptly dress again, and would often take off and put on his clothes several times before getting into bed, often ending up fully dressed. To begin with, I persisted that he undress, but later on it became too much of a struggle, so often he would just sleep with some of his clothes on. His shaving and bathing became haphazard, and he would leave a line of stubble on the back of his chin. When in the bath, he would stay briefly and splash some water over himself without washing thoroughly. His sensitivity to heat seemed to have diminished, and often he would run his bath much too hot.

During these autumn months, which would be his last at home, there were times when my intense weariness and frustration made me irritable and impatient. Often I would make excuses to get out of the house for a while—sometimes just for the luxury of making a phone call from a friend's house and feeling free to talk openly; something that I could seldom do while he was so often in the same room; able to overhear everything. If I had these times to live over again, I would try to be more patient, more tolerant, to give up some things I valued or some of my own privacy just to make his life more meaningful. Life, I have come to learn through this experience, is so short, so terribly short, and we don't know how long our times together on this earth are going to be. Opportunities lost may never occur again—we may not have a second chance. To those who read this book or go through a similar experience, I say live it to the full as much as is humanly possible; each moment is important, and our chances of giving of ourselves are limited. Though to witness a deteriorating disease like this is dreadful in every respect, remember that the grief of our lives has a meaning, too. One day, we will come to know that the crises we lived through were times when we grew the most, matured the most, in a way that doesn't happen when things are going smoothly. Above all, I have learned that to show love is most important of all. True, we are all subject to human failure and limitations, but the desire to show love and loyalty can be expressed even in small ways.

Through all this time from the beginning of the year, I had been supported by prayer from the group of six or seven women who met every Thursday together. I, too, had been one of that group and myself had learned to pray for others in need. I am convinced that prayer was the only thing that kept me from falling apart completely many times when I had to face ghastly and unexpected things and learn to accept them as reality. There is no force in the world as powerful as prayer: it overcomes the impossible time and time again. I know, because I've experienced it, that this is not an exaggeration. God is always faithful and will provide whatever is needed to get us through a crisis.

As November drew to a close, the awful realization dawned

that I would not be able physically to take care of him at home much longer. I talked to Vinton about what to do, and he suggested considering a Veterans Hospital. The closest one was at Roseburg, 172 miles away, but at that point in time I just couldn't face the wrench of him being so far away. I had not really accepted the fact of the reality of a nursing home yet—it was just a black cloud in the background—something I pushed into the back of my mind, but once again I had to force myself to look at local homes.

I remember going over to lunch with Gwen before visiting one of these homes, which had been highly recommended by a friend at church. During our lunch together, she asked about Dave, and I don't remember how the conversation went, but I broke down and sobbed my heart out. How priceless is a faithful friend. With infinite patience and understanding, Gwen supplied the comfort and strength which I needed. It was a real effort to leave the warmth of her company to go out and battle with the details that had to be faced. Somehow I made it over there and was pleasantly surprised. The staff were busy putting up Christmas decorations and greeted me with courtesy and understanding. The head nurse was busy at the moment, but if I didn't mind waiting a few minutes, she would be there. Those few minutes gave me an opportunity to look around, to soak up the atmosphere of the place, and I was impressed with what I saw. I could see that the patients were treated humanely—there was a genuine feeling of concern for their welfare. Everything was spotlessly clean, and the staff worked with cheerfulness and dedication. Mrs. Bauer turned out to be a delightful woman, more than ready to listen sympathetically and do the most she could to put me at ease. I told her that I planned to bring Dave in about the middle of January if she had a vacancy then. She made a note of this and told me to telephone her nearer the time. Her advice to me was not to visit at all during the first two weeks. In fact, she asked all relatives to do the same. It gave the staff a chance to get new patients settled in without the distractions and reminders of home. This was hard on me, she knew, but by experience she had found that it paid off. As I drove home that afternoon, a wintry sun broke through heavy clouds, sending a silver light shining across the fields and illuminating the bare, gray trunks of the trees. I remember longing so much that a light such as this could break through the clouds of Dave's life and remove its bleakness.

Some time before, Ruth and Nolan had invited us to come down to them for Christmas, and we were to leave December 21. That morning, I had to take the dogs over to the kennel, so I left Dave surrounded by our suitcases assuring him that I would be back soon. At this time, it didn't pay to tell him of plans too far in advance as he would forget so quickly, and always thought we should be leaving right away. Once at the airport, I made him sit down in the passengers' lounge while I went to get our seat assignments. While waiting in line, I made sure that he was never out of my sight, remembering the incident when he had walked away from Vinton. Fortunately, he sat quietly watching the planes taxi back and forth, and never once attempted to leave his seat. The flight down went really well; we had lunch on board and Dave obviously enjoyed himself, admiring the view of snow-capped mountains as we flew over the Cascades, and talking to his next-door neighbor. When we arrived at Oakland airport, Ruth said to me, "You look absolutely exhausted." I had not realized that I did—there wasn't much time to stop and look at myself!

It was such a relief to have the burden of responsibility now shared for this week with Ruth and Nolan and their family. It was a time of many happy reunions—our daughter Carol, from Dave's previous marriage, came over twice with her four children; Marion Johns, a long-time friend who had known Dave since childhood, and Ralph Boscacci, another boyhood friend who had grown up with him and with whom he had shared many escapades. Carol's children gave him great pleasure—he had always had a special love for children and a talent for entering into their world of thoughts and feelings. Nolan, as usual, spent much time talking to him and taking him out for drives. When he had had enough of people, he would sit in their living room quietly listening to Christmas music and seemed perfectly content there.

A large crowd of people made him more confused, and this was evident when we were sitting around the Christmas tree open-

93

ing our presents. For Dave, the meaning of receiving a gift was no longer clear. He would unwrap a present and then promptly hand it back to the giver. But I know he sensed the family atmosphere that surrounded him all that week, even though still quite reluctant to let me out of his sight.

One morning two days after Christmas, an eight-year-old boy came over to spend the day while his parents were gone. He and Dave struck up an immediate friendship and played ping pong together most of the morning. Their shouts of enthusiasm from downstairs could be clearly heard, and it was a delight to see their spontaneous enjoyment of the game and of each other's company. This was the closest to normal that I had seen him for several months. For those few hours, his handicap seemed to have dissolved completely, swallowed up by his enjoyment of the game and the stimulating company of his eight-year-old companion.

He had adjusted so well that we discussed the possibility of his staying on with Ruth and Nolan for a few days while I went home, giving me some additional free time and rest. We decided that when I left a couple of days later, Nolan would take him out for the day. We explained to him that I was going home earlier to get the dogs out of the kennel and the house ready for his return. I am not sure whether he really understood what was happening, but certainly didn't put up any opposition. I would leave on the Thursday, and he would return the following Tuesday, having been put on the plane by Ruth and Nolan with instructions to the stewardess to keep an eye on him and remind him to get off at Portland.

I really relished those four days at home alone, without the feeling that I had to be alert and in charge at all times; free to come and go without feeling guilty or that I should hurry back in case something had gone wrong. It was a real luxury. Dave missed me, they said, and would sometimes go into his room and cry, but I knew he was in the best possible hands and was so grateful for those few days free of responsibility.

The morning of his return dawned with icy roads and some fog. I called Nolan and warned him that the plane might be delayed. All went well, however, and it taxied in only a few minutes late. In spite of all we had been through that year, and the hardships still to be faced, it was a joy to see him again. There was a feeling of special closeness as we walked hand in hand out of the airport and down to the car where our little dog Star was waiting with his own unique welcome.

Nineteen seventy-seven was almost at an end. It was a year that had started out with a challenge—the challenge of seeking a solution of how to live with a hopeless diagnosis. We had tried and hoped and prayed; we had learned to accept each stage as it came. We had run the gamut of emotions from grief to hope and encouragement during those precious three months of remission. Then slowly we had slipped back from the triumph of that longed-for recovery through bitter disappointment and disillusionment to acceptance once again of the inevitable. That downturn had tested us both to the utmost. Now we had to face the fact that our lives, within a very short space of time would, of necessity, be separated.

In spite of this bleak future, we had been able to spend a joyous Christmas lived to the full, surrounded by the love and concern of those closest to us.

6. Our Separate Paths

I started the month of January, 1978 with high hopes that I would be able to cope better after our time away over Christmas and perhaps even put off admission to a nursing home for a lot longer. But four days after he came back, I wrote the following in my journal:

> He has to go into the nursing home as soon as possible be-cause I cannot cope alone any longer. I had hoped so much that I would have renewed strength after our Christmas holiday, but it seems that my stamina has almost run out, and I am right back where I started before we left for Christmas—in an exhausted state. He tries so hard to be helpful and shows love in a way he never did before, but I am so torn up inside with my own grief and the weight of the decision that I often cannot respond as I would want to. How merciful that he is receptive and open to the idea of professional help. Just how we are going to get through the next days, I have no idea; each day seems like an eter-nity of waiting, waiting, waiting. Longing for help or re-lease or relief. There is nothing more I can do—we have tried everything, so it has to be in God's hands. I know that this testing is ultimately for my growth, but I am so sick of it. It seems that there has never been a time during the last two years when I could look forward to anything.

Somehow, life does go on, even though it feels as though one is not living at all, just existing and floundering through the days like ships in a storm. Perhaps of all the times since we first had the diagnosis, this was the hardest, as not only did I have to witness his deterioration, but was carrying my own load of guilt, grief, and intense weariness. Guilt about having to put him in a nursing home, guilt about not being strong enough to take care of him any longer or find a better solution.

Thus far, I had not told him specifically that I was planning to put him in a nursing home. I just didn't know how to present it to him, as I felt sure he would refuse. What I had said was that I felt he needed more professional help than I was able to give and left it at that. Then one morning something happened which again confirmed to me that our prayers were being answered. Dave got up before I did and went out to the kitchen to make the coffee. We had a drip machine, and he had always done this first thing in the morning, and then usually brought me a cup while I was getting dressed. On this occasion, he forgot to put the carafe under the machine; he poured the water in, but there was nothing to catch it, and a flood of coffee dripped through onto the floor and all over the kitchen table. I heard the sound of dripping and rushed out to see what had happened. Sure enough, there was our coffee spreading in all directions, but not into the carafe.

Dave, realizing what he had done, turned to me and said, "Take me to a nursing home." My heart was too full to answer, but we just hugged each other silently and with deep emotion. This episode had confirmed to him that he really needed more help than I could give; wonder of wonders, he understood and realized his condition, and had asked to be taken. I then opened up and told him about the nursing homes I was considering, and he showed real interest, and seemed eager to go. "Come and see me often," he said. I wonder if perhaps the fact that he was at home alone now so much with nothing to do and no real outlet that made the nursing home seem attractive. There would be other people around him—more variety—someone to talk to at all times. Perhaps in his mind he pictured it at that moment as a place of relief for him, too? I was so touched that even in his condition, he realized that looking after him was now too much for me.

During the next two weeks, I decided we must live as fully as possible every moment. We went down to the coast one day and had lunch there. It was a stormy day with huge seas running, and out of the restaurant window we had a perfect view of the turbulent ocean, with gulls wheeling and dipping over the gray, foaming water which crashed onto the beach just below us. He enjoyed the lunch, but afterwards when I wanted him to walk on the beach with me, he was very reluctant. I did get him out and we walked quite a long way, but he was anxious to get back to the car, and we only spent about two hours actually at the beach. When I tried to get him to admire the view from a vantage point high up with a vista of the coastline stretching away to the south, he seemed frightened and couldn't focus. Perhaps the stormy sea and high cliffs were threatening to him now, as he gradually lost his sense of perspective. Once back in the car he relaxed and enjoyed the drive home, and when we got into the house said, "Where are we going now?" He had no sense of the fact that our outing for the day was finished and seemed quite disappointed.

We went to two movies, one an excellent film about ballet called *The Turning Point*. He sat quietly all through it and on this occasion, his concentration seemed to be on what he was seeing. I am sure, too, that the music helped—beautiful ballet music from Chopin and Tchaikovsky and other Russian composers. The dancing and costumes were superb, and I was so happy that he was able to enjoy this with me.

Gwen and Cliff invited us over to dinner one night, and again we were treated to some outstanding music on Cliff's stereo. I noticed that music had a very calming effect on him. It helped me, too, and lifted our spirits in a way that only music can. To me, it is far superior to words and has a language that reaches deep into the soul.

Meanwhile, I had heard nothing more from the nursing home about a vacancy, so about twice a week would call them to see if by chance something had come up. It was now January 19, and

I was close to desperation again. That morning, I decided to look at two other homes; I hated to do this because the one I had seen first was ideal and I liked the atmosphere there, but this uncertainty was devastating. Perhaps they might not have a vacancy for weeks. I remember that morning well. It was a frosty, gray January day when I set out, not convinced that I was doing the right thing, and yet . . . how much longer could we hang on?

The first home I went to had no vacancy, and I was really thankful because it didn't appeal and the surroundings were unattractive. About two miles away, set back from the street on an acre of private grounds stood the Hillview Nursing Home. As I drove in and parked the car, I paused for a minute and said a prayer. From the outside, it looked peaceful and was surrounded with lovely shrubs and trees and a big lawn. The grounds were neatly kept and across the street was a large park. I trembled as I walked up to the front door; this decision was awesome and the responsibility was mine. Once inside, I was greeted by a young aide who was sealing envelopes at the reception desk. I told her the reason for my visit, and she said she would find Mary Lindstrom, the head nurse.

While she was finding Mary, I had an opportunity to look around. The entrance hall was large and circular with a high ceiling. There was a central nurses' station, from which radiated five wings in different directions, somewhat like the spokes of a wheel. At the end of each wing was a door leading out into the grounds. The effect was spacious and pleasant. Soon, a tall, blond, attractive woman in her early thirties introduced herself as Mary Lindstrom and asked if she could show me around. The home was under new management. She was the new director of nursing services and Dick Prout was the administrator. They were just getting organized, and things were not running smoothly as yet, but she had enthusiastic plans for the future. They were not full at present, and she showed me several of the rooms. I would have liked to have had a private room for Dave, but because of the price it was out of the question. So I settled on a two-bed room. There was still some cleaning to be done on the wing where he would be, but she said they could admit him the following Monday, and would I please have him there by 9:30. I felt that since she and Dick, the administrator, were a new team just starting out, they would be likely to be trying hard to build up the home's reputation, so I decided to take the vacancy she offered. Also, my own relief at finding somewhere that would take him without additional waiting undoubtedly played a large part.

Looking back, I am not sure this was a wise decision, but in my emotional state at that time, I simply didn't have the stamina or patience to look further. I went home and told Dave the news, and mercifully he was still quite willing to go and indeed seemed eager for this new adventure. It was only fifteen minutes away from our house, so visiting would be easy. Also, Mary had not put any limits on visiting, so I would be free to come and go as often as I wanted. The relief was so great that it blotted out for the time being the separation we would have to face, and the inevitable pain this would bring. Even though I could no longer manage at home, I had not realistically faced what it would really be like when he was gone—how very final and irrevocable this move would be.

The Sunday before he went in, we had a happy reunion with Vinton and Maria, Worth and Elsa, and Arnie and Mary—three couples with whom we had been very close for several years. It was a nostalgic evening, as all three men had worked with Dave and had been loyal friends. None of us knew exactly what the future held or how it would unfold, but we were determined to make the best of it. There was a closeness between us that evening that was very special, a feeling which only comes in times of crisis.

Florence Hale, a close friend from my church, had kindly offered to drive us over to Hillview that morning of January 23, and I really welcomed the offer, as not only would it free me from driving, but I badly needed her moral support. As I finished packing his suitcase, Dave was restless, his coat on, ready to go and pacing up and down. When Florence drove in, he at once went out to greet her and was anxious to be on the way. I dared not linger over the packing or good-byes to the dogs, as I am sure that if I had weakened at that moment, the full force of what I was doing might have hit me, and we might not have made that journey to Hillview after all. Life is so strange—at times one cannot endure a moment longer; then this passes, and who knows, possibly I could have managed longer at home.

I remember making a forced effort to keep conversation flowing during that drive, mostly to hide my own anxiety and sadness, now that this move had become a reality. We were greeted at the door by Dick Prout, who took the suitcase, and then called Thelma, an aide, to come and do the admitting procedure. We went down the long corridor to Room 2, B wing. There we unpacked the suitcase, and Thelma asked me for all his medical history, what drugs he was on, who his doctor was, and finally the reason for his admission. When we got to this I took her aside into another room as I didn't want Dave to hear the details all over again. She had never heard of the disease, but listened sympathetically, and assured me she would make a point of talking to him every day and checking on his needs. I could see that she had real compassion and dedication. Dave, meanwhile, was in his room sitting on the bed, apparently quite unconcerned. Up to now he had taken the whole thing in his stride and seemed to be enjoying the change and new surroundings.

After the admission form was filled out, we walked back to the main entrance where Florence was waiting. Now came the hardest part; now we would have to say good-bye; this was the first day of a new life for us both. Still, Dave didn't realize exactly what had happened. He came to the door with us, but made no attempt to leave when we did, and quite happily turned back in again. I looked around and saw him, still with his coat on, waving good-bye just as though we would soon be back. I felt quite numb and overwhelmed by how cooperative he had been. It had been almost too easy; I had braced myself for tears and emotion, and he had accepted the whole thing in complete trust. Florence came in and we talked for a while after returning home; I was so dazed that first day that the reality didn't register, and although I was tired, it was impossible to sleep.

It was not until the following day that the new situation began to be felt. Mostly, it was wondering how he was doing now, were they being kind to him, were they trying to understand, how soon will it be safe to visit? I wonder how he slept last night? I got through that first day by keeping busy, trying to catch up on many things I had not been free to do while he was still at home.

The second day the pain was excruciating. Somehow he got to a telephone that evening—his second day in the home—and called me. It was a nightmare. "Can you come and pick me up?" he asked.

Never before had I had to refuse him. "Dave, I can't do that, but I'll be over to see you very soon." He couldn't understand why I was not willing to go over and get him at once. Later that day, I called to see how he was doing and one of the nurses answered; he was having adjustment problems, she said. I asked if I could speak to him. He was evidently close by, and when he picked up the phone, I could hear him sobbing. I can't remember what I said, but it can't have been much help to him. I sobbed myself afterwards, the kind of crying that is the only way to express the agony I felt—agony for myself and for him and for the blackness of life; for the desolation of our lives that were now separated; for the loneliness and grief; for all the "Might have beens" and the "If onlys." The situation was made worse later that afternoon when the original nursing home I had contacted called to say they now had a vacancy. If only I had waited two days longer. The feeling of guilt was indescribable. The rest of that day was a blur of pain, tears, and remorse. Since he was having a hard time settling in, Mary Lindstrom suggested that I not come over to see him until Friday, at the earliest. Each day I talked to her on the phone, and thankfully, the following day, he was doing a bit better. I told her that he had called me, and warned her to watch out for this. Nevertheless, a day or two later, he asked one of the other patients to call his home number, and ask me if I could come and take him home. I explained as best I could that he could not come home and having to say this was perhaps one of the worst experiences I have ever lived through. It cannot be expressed in words.

Friday, January 27, I went over to visit for the first time, and took him out to lunch. He was not in the hall when I came in, so I went down to his room, and he was sitting on the bed, fully dressed, with his coat on and a kind of dazed expression. When he saw me, he rushed up and hugged me with tears in his eyes. "I thought you were never going to come," he said. We sat down and talked for a while and I did my best to reassure him. The aide, Thelma, who had filled out his admission form, was going to lunch, too, just as we were about to leave, and offered to take us in her car. It went off well, and he relaxed and enjoyed the outing and our company. I dreaded the return, not knowing how he would react to having to go back in to the home. But there was no problem; he followed me in without any opposition. Although he was in a two-bed room, at that time there was not another patient in the extra bed, so he had the room to himself. I felt relieved that this was so; he had his own private bathroom, and I had brought pictures and some flowers to make the room more cheerful. It looked out on the back lawn beyond which was a bank planted with tall trees and shrubs, so his view was private and peaceful. From then on I would visit him every Tuesday and Friday; quite often on Sundays, too, and we would go out for a meal and a drive. Usually, I brought Star with me, and we would walk in the grounds before I left. To begin with, Dave was exceptionally good about going back in after we had been out for a drive. Each time we pulled into that parking lot after an outing, I dreaded the separation that must inevitably come. I wondered so much how he really felt; he was so obedient, so anxious to cooperate, and for quite a long time, he didn't even ask to be taken home. He seemed to understand that he must be there, and should make the best of it.

One Sunday afternoon when I came over, he was so busy talking to one of the older patients and helping her to walk, that he hardly noticed when I left. Times like these made it easier for me. The activities director, Shirley, did her best to keep him occupied. She had him working with clay models and one day he did quite well, but his attention span was a problem. She would gather a group of patients in the activity room each morning and read the paper to them. Then followed a discussion of current events. Shirley was young and vivacious and seemed to relate well to most of the patients, as her enthusiasm was infectious—her liking for and patience with older people was genuine.

The aide, Thelma, was very consistent and made it a point to spend some time talking to Dave each day. When she knew I was coming over, she would always have him ready to leave, shaved and in clean clothes. The laundry was a major source of frustration. I had told the staff that I would take his clothes home and wash them myself, but often the message didn't get through and they would go into the hospital laundry, which ruined most clothes because of high water temperatures. So each time I came in, I would check his room thoroughly, and put aside the things I wanted to take home to wash. Also, in his confused state, he wasn't responsible for what happened to his clothes, and would often leave his shoes or socks in another patient's room. It was quite common for clothes to disappear—the aides were poorly paid and the temptation was too much for some of them. In Dave's case, I decided not to leave any good-quality clothes in his closet, but kept them at home and brought over his good clothes for special outings. We were fortunate in that the only thing we lost was a jacket which matched his jeans; it disappeared without a trace. I told Mary about this, and she assured me she would follow up on it, but I am not sure that she did.

After he had been there about three weeks, he made friends with "Grandma," a patient who had broken her hip just before Christmas and was in for convalescence and therapy. Her room was across the corridor from his and she enjoyed company. Often two or three patients would be in her room each evening watching television, with Grandma holding court and enjoying every minute of it. Her daughter, Kathy, came over to see her every day and both of them took Dave under their wing.

Quite often, if it wasn't my day for a visit, Kathy would take him out to lunch. I was so grateful for this and for the fact that they both liked him, so were able to help each other mutually. Grandma had a sharp tongue, but was good-hearted. She could be counted on to speak her mind and you knew it was the truth— she was incapable of pretense! I developed a real friendship with Kathy and admired her dedication to her mother and her compassion for Dave. She was also good to the other patients, and always took time to chat with those who were sitting in the hall when she came in.

As time went on, the four of us would go out to lunch together, Grandma with her wheelchair, which had to be folded up and put in the back of the car, but she managed well and made the most of the attention she drew at restaurants with her handicap. She was sharp-witted and observant, often humorous, though frequently at someone else's expense.

Mary had a problem getting adequate staff; as mentioned before, the wage for a nurses' aide is minimal, and so attracts poor-caliber people most of the time. No training or experience is required, and the work is heavy, unrewarding, and often distasteful. Unless the head nurse can really provide incentives and direction, the quality of care suffers and "difficult" patients are often neglected or get inadequate attention. My impression of Mary was that she was compassionate, but inexperienced so far as running a home of this size was concerned. There were ninety-five beds on the five wings, and the home had been allowed to deteriorate under the former management, so she had a big job ahead of her. She seemed more comfortable in her office than out on the floor, and undoubtedly had all the book learning necessary, but lacked experience in delegating responsibility and enforcing discipline. She was conscientious about the food, which had been very poor to begin with, and took a lot of trouble finding an experienced chef and checking the patients' meals to see that they were appetizing.

In mid-March, Dick Prout called me one day to say that the wing Dave was on had been assigned by the state inspector to welfare patients, and that they would have to move Dave into a four-bed room. For two months now, he had been in his own room alone, which I think suited him, and I dreaded the thought of putting him with three other patients just after he was beginning to settle in. Dick explained that he could stay in his present room, but we would have to pay ten dollars a day extra, bringing our monthly bill to about one thousand dollars or more. Reluctantly, I agreed to the move on condition that as soon as there was a two-bed room available, he would be moved into it. The four-bed room was not nearly so nice, even though there was a divider between the four beds which gave some measure of privacy. The bathroom was at the end farthest away from Dave's bed, as was also his clothes closet, so it was awkward and sometimes embarrassing for him to use it because of disturbing the other patients. Fortunately, his neighbor, Fred, was a nice, quiet man—he was there for some neurological problem and apparently had no family close by to take care of him.

Easter came early that year, at the end of March, and I decided that I would take Dave to the sunrise service which we had been to several times before, with Worth and Elsa Bellamy. It would mean picking him up at about six A.M., so I gave Mary instructions to pass on to the night staff to have him dressed and ready when I arrived. As it turned out, that Saturday night there was only one aide and one R.N. on duty; the others had either not bothered to show up or had called in sick, as it was a holiday weekend. That night, too, one of the patients died, so the two on duty had far more than they could handle adequately. Upon my arrival, Dave was still sound asleep in bed; one of the women patients was wandering around in the nude with the male aide frantically trying to coax her back into her room. He was acutely embarrassed when I appeared on the scene, and apologized profusely to me, explaining about their hectic night. Since we were late already, I asked him if he could help me by shaving Dave, but he said no. I couldn't understand why—either he was too busy, or else he was afraid of Dave and didn't know how to handle him. He was groggy with sleep still, and it took longer than usual to get him dressed, as if I tried to hurry, he just got more confused. He was amazingly patient with our fumbling efforts to get his clothes on.

That was a nostalgic Easter morning. I remembered the other, happier years when we had gone to this service together and all that it had meant; it was hard not to cry during the beautiful, moving service with massed choirs singing all the familiar Easter hymns. Dave sat quietly through most of it, but occasionally would reach out with his hand as though to touch the person in front of him—I imagine he was hallucinating. He looked gaunt and thin that morning, and the days' growth of beard on his chin didn't help. The progress of the disease plus the major adjustment of the last two months were all the more noticeable now when he was away from the home. Most likely, there were times when he didn't eat properly because they wouldn't take the time to supervise him at meals.

I was glad that we made the effort to go as he was delighted to see Worth and Elsa and chatted away with Worth as he always had in the past. We stopped at Denny's for breakfast after the service and it felt so good to have him back with friends again even for those few hours, sharing a day that meant a lot to all of us.

The sun broke through after we got back to Hillview, and we spent some time outside in the grounds enjoying this lovely morning. Later, Kathy brought her mother out in the wheelchair, and I stayed with them until about noon. I felt that, all in all, it had been a triumphant Easter, the best we could have spent under the circumstances.

My life at home often held times of acute loneliness and emptiness; no matter what I was doing during the day, my mind was mostly with him, looking forward to my next visit. The time of day when it was worst was always between five and seven in the evening—dinnertime. Eating alone seemed so meaningless, and there is a dreadful void about that time of the day; even now, three years later, I still dislike this time of day. The feeling of guilt was still very strong, and it takes a long time for these scars to heal. When our lives were disrupted by this enforced separation, part of me died, too. I am sure that anyone who has gone through the same experience will understand what I mean. One will never be quite the same again because a phase of life—a chapter of existence— has ended. In our case, it was so final, and I knew deep down that he would not be able to come home again. Often I agonized as to whether I should bring him home for a few hours, but would this have been kind or cruel? Would he have wanted to stay, and would there have been a major scene trying to get him back to Hillview? I pondered these questions, and felt that our lives were disrupted enough without the risk of another painful event. So I never did bring him back, and I still have mixed feelings about this.

In early April, Grandma had recovered enough to be sent home. I am sure that Dave, as well as many of the other patients, missed her. She had really seemed to enjoy the company at the nursing home, and most of the time was the life and soul of the party with her quick-witted remarks. About a week later, Kathy and I planned that we would all meet for lunch at Roses', a Jewish restaurant on the northwest side of town. It was a Monday morning, and I went over to get Dave about 10:30, allowing some extra time in case he needed help with dressing. As I walked down the hall to E wing, the smell was overpowering. To my horror, I discovered that it was indeed coming from his room. With a sinking heart, I walked in and found him sitting on the bed fully dressed. He had had violent diarrhea and was just sitting there, seemingly not knowing what to do or how to ask for help. I am sure the accident happened because he was too embarrassed to go to the bathroom—inconvenient as it was—and waited too long.

There was no sign of any nurse or aide on that wing; everyone seemed to have disappeared, and I am sure they were avoiding that room for as long as possible.

In a fury, I stormed into Mary's office and told her. She came out to the nurses' station, but the R.N. in charge was out for a coffee break. She then went down the wing and found the aide, Pat, who was on duty. Pat was new that morning; she was a tall, raw-boned, raucous girl, with a rough, offhand manner. When Nancy told her to come at once and clean Dave up, I could see it was the last thing she wanted to do. However, she came reluctantly, but was not much help at all, and Dave obviously disliked her. He must have had a badly upset stomach, as he had also vomited into the dish on his bedside table, and this had not been cleaned up.

I felt nauseated by this event, and it really took the edge off our lunch party. I asked Dave if he felt like eating, and he seemed to be all right, but I was afraid all through lunch of a recurrence of his upset stomach. This stands out in my mind as one of the worst things I had to deal with at Hillview. The incredible indifference to a patient in this condition, with no one attempting to do anything about it until I got there, is hard to understand. Inevitably, the blame has to lie with Mary; if she had been a strong and directive head nurse, she would have dealt with this at once, or told one of the aides to clean him up. I was aware that they were short of staff that morning, but instead of sitting in her office, she could have helped on that wing where the need was greatest.

This led to a discussion with Vinton as to whether we would leave him at Hillview, or move him to another home. At about this time, four different people suggested to me that he would get much better care in a veterans' hospital. We had to go in for a routine checkup with Dr. Sanger, and as we were leaving he said, "You know, the V.A. should really be taking care of him, not the nursing home." Then Kathy, whose husband had been in the veterans' hospital at Roseburg, suggested the same thing and encouraged me to pursue it further. Third, Lee, a male aide who was very mature and had been in the service himself, told me that his case would be much better understood at a V.A. hospital.

The fourth person was Vinton, who had already suggested this alternative several months before, at a time when I was not ready for him to be so far away from home. Our physician, Dr. Masenhimer, had transferred to the V.A. in Roseburg some three years before, so I decided to go down and talk to him about the possibility of getting Dave in.

Kathy kindly offered to come down with me, and it was a great help having her company on the long 172-mile drive. Our appointment was not until 3:45, so we left home about eleven and stopped on the way for lunch. Dr. Masenhimer told me what the procedure would be: we would have to send in an application giving his full medical history and the neurologist's latest report. This would be considered by the admissions committee, and if accepted, his name would be placed on their waiting list.

Probably, he would be on Ward 6—a psychiatric ward—until they decided whether he would benefit from any therapy they could give. As we drove home, I realized that I was still resisting the idea of having him so far away. I had grown used to seeing him two or three times a week, and the thought of putting this distance between us really hurt. True, he would have much better care, but did that outweigh the benefits of my being able to see him twice a week? Would he ever remember me if I could only see him two or three times a month? How would the upheaval of another change affect him? I mulled all these questions over with Kathy on the way home, and she was positive that this was the best way to go. She didn't pressure me, but presented the facts and left the final decision up to me.

Deep down, I dreaded another more drastic separation, pointing again to the fact that we would have less and less time together in the future. The times we had together now were very precious; I lived for the days when I could take him out and reassure him that I still cared. About a week after our trip to Roseburg, I finally decided that I would go ahead with the Roseburg plan. I contacted Dr. Sanger and told him that I would like him to send the medical information down to the V.A. with a view to his admission as soon as they had a vacancy. I also had to realize that my responsibility was to do what was best for him, since he could not decide for himself—above all, this was more important than my feelings.

Often, good-byes at the nursing home would be difficult now. Sometimes he would balk when he had to go in, and then came the painful decision as to whether or not to say good-bye, or just slip away when he was preoccupied with something else. Most often, I chose the latter course. His memory was so short now that mercifully he would soon forget me after I left. But if I made a point of saying good-bye, he would pursue me down the hall and try to come out to the car with me. On several occasions, I left quickly when he was talking to somebody else, only to find that he had seen me and came running down the wing asking if he could come, too. At this time, I had a part-time job, so I told him I had to leave in time to get to work. Nevertheless, it was extremely painful, and often I felt as though I had betrayed him. I can remember many times when I drove home in tears, and an equal number of times when I set out for Hillview in an agony of anticipation as to what I might find when I got there.

Frequently, he would not only be unshaved, but would have dressed himself without any supervision; two or three shirts one on top of the other, or back to front; odd socks or none at all; odd shoes or no shoes. Alzheimer patients cannot keep track of any of their belongings so often I would find some of his clothes or shoes in another patient's room or closet. Sometimes, he would wander into the shower room and leave his shoes there. Always in his bedside drawer was a collection of odds and ends such as bottle caps, pieces of string, rolled-up pieces of paper, toothpicks, chewing gum wrappers, shoelaces—everything under the sun seemed to end up in that drawer, and I was constantly cleaning it out. I soon learned to look under the bed as well if something was missing.

Early in May, I decided I would take him out and spend a night at a motel to give him a change and spend some more time with him. When I arrived that evening to pick him up, Dee, the R.N. on duty, said that he had been rowdy and hostile that day, and gave me some tranquilizers to take with me in case I had any trouble. We had a very nice, leisurely dinner at a restaurant which overlooked an indoor ice rink, so we watched the skaters for some time after finishing our dinner. He was in a relaxed mood and at times was almost normal in his responses. When we arrived at the motel, he became anxious and confused and kept saying: "We've got to catch that plane to San Francisco." This outing probably brought back to him times when he was travelling, and San Francisco was a town he had always loved. We watched a TV program, and soon after he became sleepy. No doubt they had given him a tranquilizer before he left, so we went to bed about nine, and he slept soundly, only waking up once in the night.

Early next morning as we lay there together, I watched him and he looked so at peace, still sound asleep. I wished so much we could both die at this moment, that time would stand still and we wouldn't have to move on into another day of struggle and pain into a future which we knew was hopeless. Oh, God, how

111

I wish you would take us both now to be with you, so that we wouldn't have to travel the rest of this journey.

We don't know how long it will go on—only you know that, and only you know the meaning to all of this. So we have to brace ourselves and get on with the business of living and leave all the outcomes to you.

We took a long time getting ready to leave. I helped Dave with his bath and shaving, and then he said what I had dreaded: "Let's go home." I said, "We're going to have breakfast first." I couldn't say any more than that. He was in a restless, anxious mood at breakfast, and then when I drove him back to Hillview about ten o'clock, he was disgusted with me. It really hurt having to leave him there, looking so nice; clean and shaved. What would his day hold, I wondered? I hoped that the memory of our night out together would somehow stay in his memory and give him comfort and reassurance that he was not forgotten.

As the weather improved, I would often bring a picnic lunch which we would take into the park. I always brought Star with me, and it was touching to see how exuberantly he greeted Dave each time—jumping up into his lap and licking his face in greeting. For those two or three hours, we could forget the home and just resume our lives together, trying to live in the present moment without thinking of the past or the future. Each Friday, we would go to a Loaves and Fishes luncheon which was held at a church nearby, taking with us four or five of the other patients who were well enough to go. The food was always good and to begin with, I think Dave enjoyed these outings. At least it was a break in his routine and something different to look forward to. Quite often, he would help me with the other patients, assisting them in and out of the car, so was able to feel useful in this way.

About the second week in June, he became very restless one Friday at the luncheon. He had finished eating long before anyone else and kept saying he wanted to go, which was impossible because the others were still eating and could not be hurried. If only his attention span had been long enough, he could have played cards, dominoes, or checkers, as often many of those who came would stay afterwards and enjoy card games or bingo. It was embarrassing for me, because he paced up and down, repeatedly asking to leave and became quite angry and disruptive when I refused. Regretfully, I knew the time was at an end for these luncheons. If he was going to behave like this, it was no pleasure to him or the other patients.

The new activities director, Jerry Rosemeyer, had organized a different event for the following Friday. We were going out to Sauvie Island, a large island in the Columbia river, for a picnic, weather permitting. There would be a large gathering from all over the Portland area from different nursing homes, and a catered lunch was to be served. There was also fishing in the Columbia for those who were interested. It was a great opportunity for me to take him out for almost the entire day, as we were due to leave at 9:30. To begin with, he was not too enthusiastic about the idea—I think it was the unknown which disturbed him—but we set off with Star and the son of one of the patients at Hillview, Bob Fletcher. I was glad to have him in the car with us, in case Dave became restless or unmanageable. Although the day was fun for me, I don't think he really enjoyed it. He had no interest at all in the fishing (something he had really enjoyed as a boy), and when I tried to take him for a walk, he seemed uncertain and fearful. I expect he was afraid of this unfamiliar territory, for by now he had reached the stage where well-known surroundings were important. He may have thought that we would get lost, and once again I noticed that a large crowd of people put him on edge. When our picnic lunch arrived, he was given a paper plate and we had to stand in line to get our food which was served from a long table. He didn't want to sit at a table with several of the others, so we went and had our lunch in the car. After he had finished, he fidgeted with his paper plate, kept folding and unfolding it, and when I got home I found it neatly folded under the car mat! He seemed most secure in the car, and spent most of the afternoon there, while I kept an eye on him between short walks with Star over to the river to see how the fishermen were doing. He was relieved when, at about three o'clock, it was time to leave and we drove back to Hillview.

113

At that time, I had not realized that he was beginning to reach the point when the outings I thought would be fun for him were in fact not so, because strange places, even when he was accompanied by me, may have been threatening to him. I know now that this is true of most Alzheimer patients—they have lost the capacity to recognize where they are, so an outing to a place which even once may have been familiar, seems risky and uncomfortable. This kind of day, then, was in fact more fun for me than for him.

My sister, Helen, was coming to visit me and was due to arrive on June 24 by Pan Am from London. It was such a joy to have her with me for two and a half weeks. It broke my pattern of loneliness and meaninglessness at home and gave life a purpose again. Two days after she arrived, we went over to see Dave. It was a perfect June day, so we packed a picnic lunch and took Star with us. On the way over, I remember a nagging fear about how I would find him—a fear that had become all too familiar during these last months. Would he be shaved and clean? Or would I have to shave and dress him myself? Who would be on duty? Will I find his room in a mess, with his clothes scattered on the bed or in somebody else's closet?

I came in at the back entrance and walked down C wing to the front hall. It was about 11:00 A.M. and things looked relatively peaceful and under control; the floor had been freshly waxed and polished; most of the patients were dressed and looked clean. They had come to know me well, and usually I would stop on my way to Dave's room to say hello to the ones I knew the best, especially those who had befriended Dave—two in particular: Audrey Bailey and Elizabeth Campbell.

He was wandering aimlessly up and down outside his room on E wing. He looked sallow and drawn, had two days' growth of beard and his hair was uncombed and bushy; it was also much too long as the barber had not been in lately. With a sinking heart, I took him into the bathroom to shave him. He was glad to see me but seemed dopey and out of touch. His eyes were blank and expressionless. It took me some time to find his razor, comb, brush, and towel, but finally we got started. Shaving him

114

was difficult that day and took much longer than usual; also I was so upset at seeing him this way when I had wanted him to look especially good for Helen that I didn't do a very good job myself. I called in on Mary on our way out to the car, and she told me that yesterday he had had a bad day. He had been very restless and was pacing until late at night; when they tried to get him into bed he resisted and became angry, disturbing some of the other patients. So they gave him a stiff dose of Haldol which had knocked him out until about nine this morning. I told her that I was shocked at his appearance, and she apologized, saying it was the only way they knew to handle him. The other patients had to be considered, too.

Gradually, the fresh air and good food helped him—he recognized Helen and his face lit up when he saw her. We kept him out as long as possible and gave him a good walk in the park, and he gradually became less distraught. Helen wanted to take some photographs, and it was difficult to get him to stand still and look at the camera, although he did eventually stand long enough for her to get a picture, but his head was down looking at his hands. I know she was horrified to see him in this condition and so was I. I told her that it was by far the worst he had ever been, and it was unfortunate that it had to coincide with her first visit to Hillview.

I went more thoroughly into the whole situation with Mary, and she told me that often his restlessness was worse on a Sunday if I didn't come over and there was little or nothing to keep him occupied. They were usually short-staffed, especially on the night shift. He was noticeably better after I had taken him out, so after this I made a point of always giving him a long walk and keeping him out longer, so that he would be tired enough to settle down at night.

I know it was hard for Helen to cope with the trauma of the nursing home. She would wait outside while I went in to get Dave, and was upset by what she saw there. True, it is a depressing sight to see a number of patients in their wheelchairs, just sitting, with nobody to talk to, and most likely no visitors. They are put away and forgotten in many instances, so are entirely dependent on the attentions of the staff, which often leaves much to be desired.

Towards the end of Helen's stay, we had planned to go to a horse show which would be an all-day event. We debated whether or not to take Dave. I really would have liked to take him, but on the basis of past experience doubted very much whether he would be able to concentrate and sit for that length of time. So I went to Hillview for a couple of hours to take him out before we left. Audrey Bailey was sitting with him when I arrived. "How thankful I am that you've come," she said, as Dave immediately rushed up and took my hand. Audrey told me that he had been having a bad morning, tense and unhappy. She had tried to make a point of staying with him as much as possible. We left and went for our usual walk and picnic lunch. He was quite relaxed and seemed at peace as we sat on one of the park benches, talking together about Helen, about his family, and what we might do on our next outing. I had promised to be back to take Helen to the horse show by 2:30 that afternoon, so our time was limited, and with sadness I realized that it was drawing to a close. I had much inner conflict that day between my loyalty to Dave and my loyalty to Helen. At that moment, if I had had the choice between staying with him longer, I would have done so, because he really seemed to need me that day. On the other hand, Helen would be with me for only a week longer, so which was the right priority?

After our return to Hillview, I quietly asked one of the nurses and Audrey to distract him while I left, but today this wasn't going to be easy. He was watching me, and when I started to walk down to the back door, he ran after me, begging me to take him too. These are agonizing moments. I tried to explain that I had promised to take Helen to the show—that we would be there all afternoon and he would probably find it boring. How lame are the excuses one makes under these kind of conditions! "Why can't I go, too?" he asked. "Not this time, Dave," I answered. He became angry and turned away with a disgusted expression on his face.

I left that day with my heart in turmoil—had I been selfish

in wanting Helen to myself for the rest of the day? Certainly, I felt guilty about this decision; I was adding extra pain to his life that day, something I would have avoided at all costs. There were many instances of just this kind of thing during those months at the nursing home—times when I left in tears, hating myself, my responsibility, the rending pain of seeing his condition, his dependence, and sometimes having to deny his requests.

On July 12, when Helen left to fly back to England, we decided it would be a nice outing for him to go to the airport with us to see her off. Vinton kindly offered to come too, and we left that afternoon about 2:00 P.M. It was a really hot day, and so long as we were in the car, Dave did fairly well. We went into the airport restaurant for a snack and a cool drink, and then gathered in the departure lounge waiting for the announcement to board. The 747 taxied in, majestic and enormous, its blue and silver colors glistening in the sunlight. A lump rose in my throat as it came time to say good-bye; Helen was having difficulty, too. She hugged me with tears in her eyes, and then turned to Dave and held him for a moment, "Good-bye, Dave." It was too much—the tears were now streaming down her cheeks as she walked out to join the long line filing on board. She was unable to look back and I understood why. Later she wrote and apologized because she didn't feel she had said good-bye properly. There was no need of an apology because her expression had said everything she felt but could not express in words.

Toward the end of July, I had an inner feeling—it seemed like a sort of message—that Dave would not be at Hillview much longer. We had heard in June from the V.A. Hospital that he was on their waiting list, and they expected it would be about three months before a vacancy became available. I racked my brains for different things to do with him other than just lunch and a walk and thought it might be a good idea to try the zoo, as he had always liked animals. As the afternoons were hot now, I set out early in the morning, having called to tell them to have him cleaned up and ready to go. Pat was on duty that day—worse luck—and told me in sugary tones that she had got him all ready for me. To my horror I saw that his jeans were stained

117

and his shirt rumpled as though he had slept in it. There wasn't time to go through the whole rigmarole of changing his clothes again, so I left him as he was. It wasn't a very good expedition. To begin with, he hardly looked at the animals at all, and wanted to keep moving. The giraffes were about the only thing that caught his attention. I tried to keep him there as long as I could in the hope that he would settle and get some pleasure out of it, but once more he seemed glad to get back to the car.

We stopped at a crowded restaurant for lunch; one of the worst meals I've ever eaten. After I'd paid the bill, I had to go to the ladies' room and told Dave to wait for me by the cash-register desk. There was a seat just inside the door, but with all the comings and goings I felt doubtful if he would stay. I was in and out of the ladies' room in a flash, my mind on Dave. Sure enough, he was not sitting by the desk, but was outside, fortunately not too far away.

A major problem now in restaurants was when he had to go to the men's room. On one occasion he went in and I waited for about ten minutes, becoming more uncomfortable by the second. It was fairly late in the evening, so I chose my moment and cautiously went in to see what was happening. He was standing staring into the mirror; he had washed off his face and his hair was wet, but whether he went to the bathroom or not remains a mystery. I believe what happened is that when he got in there, he would forget how to get out again. During the course of two years or so, I have rushed into more men's rooms than anyone would believe! In time, I came to ignore the surprised and shocked glances of other male occupants and would try a short explanation instead. Even our worst moments sometimes have a humorous side!

During the hot August weather, I went to Hillview more often in the evenings; sometimes we would go out to dinner and then have a walk afterwards—other times I would drop over later with one of the dogs, take him into the park, and we would usually end up at the Dairy Queen for a milkshake or a cool drink. He recognized the road back quite well now, and always when we got to that fatal turn just before the entrance, he would show his disgust and reluctance at having to go in again. It's an experience I hope I never have to go through again: that dreadful feeling inside of betrayal, of knowing how he must feel, is beyond description. I have been fortunate enough never to suffer severe physical pain or illness, but emotional pain is just as real, just as devastating.

Looking back on those days, I don't know how I made it through the many sad partings. It was as though the fabric of our lives had been torn into shreds, into a meaningless jumble of meeting and parting, yet it did have meaning, I am sure. I asked Mary how long it took him to settle down after I had left. She told me that in the beginning, it had been difficult—he would often cry and be upset for several hours. As time went on, however, he would forget more quickly, and it was easier to distract his thoughts with the help of another patient or one of the nurses. I was thankful to hear this and it made the burden a little lighter for me.

One evening after dinner we were walking in the park, when suddenly a little bird fluttered down out of nowhere and settled on Dave's head. It was twittering happily and was not the least afraid. Then it fluttered off his head and onto a nearby fence, where it continued its song, almost as though it was trying to tell us something. We were both surprised but delighted by this little messenger, who seemed to have been sent to give us special cheer, reassuring us that all was well and we were not forgotten.

Toward the end of August, Mary warned me that they would not be able to keep Dave much longer. His restlessness and hostility toward some of the staff had made them afraid to handle him. One aide, Betty, had refused to have anything to do with him because of his unpredictable moods. He had not actually hit anyone, but had threatened to. On one occasion during Mary's vacation, he had not been shaved for a week and when I asked the reason why, was told that he wanted to grow a beard. Twice during that week I had specifically asked that he be shaved, but with no results. The story about the beard was, I am sure, an excuse because no one wanted to do it. I am sure that by this time he knew just how to manipulate them or play angry so

119

as to put them off. Perhaps it was the only way he could assert himself with his other faculties fast dwindling.

Mary asked me if I had heard anything from the V.A. hospital yet about his admission, but I told her that I hadn't. She then suggested that to speed things up, it might be a good idea for Dr. Baker, the Hillview doctor, to write up a report on Dave and send it to the V.A., telling them about his unmanageable behavior. If there was no response to this, she told me that I would have to find another home or hospital willing to take him. Another crisis to face, and I had planned to go down for a week to see Ruth and Nolan starting September 5. Naturally, it was not easy to leave with all this going on in the background. On September 1, 1978, I wrote the following prayer in my journal:

O Lord, today the pain is very deep—like a sharp sword—like having my insides eaten away. I wish that this pain I suffer, these tears I shed, could somehow be used constructively, above all to reassure and comfort Dave, to create in him a knowledge of your presence. I commit this pain to you, since nothing committed to you is ever wasted, and I trust you to use it in the mysterious way you work, to bring about beauty, truth, and love.

You came to this earth that we "might have life and have it abundantly," and I thank you for that promise and for the love and support you have always provided in my life, even when I was unaware of it. I know, mentally, that you never fail, even though sometimes it seems, because we are so limited to visible signs, that you have forsaken us. I also know that there must be reasons why you allow us to live on the brink of the precipice, as it were at certain times.

I am writing this because I so desperately want to find the meaning to this suffering. I am convinced that it was never your will that we should live in a state of sickness, disease, broken relationships, accidental death, and so on, the list could go on indefinitely. But how do we distinguish between the things you allow to happen, and those that happen through human error, neglect, or rebellion?

I hope that what I am seeking is light to guide me through a very dark valley, but sometimes in the midst of trouble my own motives are not clear as my suffering is so closely bound to Dave's. At this point, I don't know how to pray at all except to cling to you in utter helplessness.

On Monday, September 4, which was Labor Day, I went over and took Dave out for a long drive. We started out with lunch at the Greenwood Inn, and then drove all 'round Portland, all the familiar places where he had audited with his boss, Worth, the parks and streets that he had known so well. I wanted to get him away for as long as possible, hoping that he might settle down better that night and not give them any trouble.

We ended up with a long walk in the park, and then I sat and talked with him and two of the other patients before leaving. Audrey, as usual, was most helpful, and when I left called him over to talk to her, thereby making the good-bye less painful.

The morning I was due to leave for California, I felt uneasy about him and called to find out how things were. He had had a good night's rest; in fact had slept late, which was what I had hoped for. Sue, the R.N. in charge, told me not to worry, that they would take good care of him while I was gone. I heard nothing from Hillview the week that I was away, so assumed that all was well.

The day after my return, I went over to see him again, and was in his room sorting out some clothes when Mary appeared at the door. When we got back from lunch, she would like to talk to me. I decided to enjoy our time out together, whatever Mary's news might be, and didn't hurry to get back. I was sure it had something to do with his admission to the V.A. Hospital. She told me that on the basis of Dr. Baker's information they had agreed to admit Dave on Monday, September 18. It was almost too good to believe and had happened so quickly, much more quickly than I had ever dreamed possible. Mary had talked to the admissions director, Mr. House, and I was to confirm this arrangement with him.

While I was away, Dave had walked out of the home one evening and slipped away unnoticed. I have since thought that perhaps they didn't really care any more and were even relieved when he disappeared. Mercifully, one of the evening shift, Dee, on her way to work, saw him. He was about four miles away, walking fast in the direction of Portland, and at first when she stopped and spoke to him, he looked scared and tried to avoid her. When he realized who she was, he consented to let her take him back.

My feelings of thankfulness that his time at Hillview was now almost over can only be imagined. There were only three days left to prepare for the move to Roseburg. I called Mr. House, and confirmed that we would be down on Monday and asked which building to come to for admission. It would be on the second floor of building 2, he told me, and to be sure and bring all his medical records. I decided to take him out of the home Sunday afternoon; we would then go and spend the night in Salem, which would make our drive an hour shorter the next day.

It had been almost exactly eight months since we left home that foggy January morning to begin a separation brought about by a tragic necessity, something that neither of us had ever dreamed of. It was an unsatisfactory alternative, but the choices were so limited. If it had not been for the V.A. hospital, I would have had to consider putting him in a mental hospital—an equally dreadful solution. For Alzheimer patients the choices are still very limited. On the whole, nursing staffs have not been trained to understand them, and it takes special qualities of patience and dedication to deal with them. Kindness and imagination are so very important when handling these patients. I believe that the dedicated members of the staff at Hillview did try their best to meet his needs. I am thankful, too, for the patients who took him under their wing: Audrey Bailey, Elizabeth Campbell, Kathy Jones and her mother.

Thus, the first phase of our separation ended. I realized full well that this could be the last time he would be close by. I was going to have to face the fact of a long drive now when I visited, and a night or two away from home. I didn't know how I was going to tell him where he was going, but I'd do it somehow. I'd just have to trust that this was for the best. The part I played in his life would inevitably be smaller now because of distance. I wondered if he would remember me as time went on.

7. Walking the Precipice at Roseburg

Sunday, September 17, 1978: We are on the brink of another major change; I have mixed feelings of relief, yet regret that he will have to be so far away—there is something so very final about a distance of 172 miles. I had planned to go over to Hillview and pick Dave up about 2:00 P.M., but decided to leave earlier as I had to do his packing and clean up his room. When I arrived, Dave was out. Worth and Elsa had come over unexpectedly after church, and had taken him to lunch. This made his packing easier for me as he wasn't hovering in the background, continually asking when we could go or distracting me in other ways.

When they returned from lunch, Dave was in excellent spirits and all the more so when he saw me. I was thankful that he wouldn't have to spend any more time here; it was getting to the point where the staff had just about given up on him and he had completely outgrown the kind of care they were able to give. I felt sorry that this era at the nursing home had to be. If I could have found more adequate help at home, I am sure I could have managed until we could get a vacancy at the V.A. Hospital. However, that is water under the bridge now, and even the nursing home had its good moments. It is so easy in retrospect to remember only the painful times without acknowledging the good as well. It was a phase of our lives that we had to go through, and perhaps its main value was in preparing us for the more lengthy, distant separation that was to follow.

As we said our final farewells and went out to the car, the sky, which had been steadily darkening for some time, resounded with a clap of thunder bringing on a downpour. As we drove out from Hillview, streams of water were coursing down the driveway.

Dave, as usual, entered into the spirit of the outing. I told him we were going to Salem to spend the night there in a motel and would have dinner with Vint and Maria. I felt a surge of happiness at being able to have this night with him—a precious twenty-four hours or so when our lives would be together. It felt like a privilege, a gift, to be able to do this. We checked in at the Holiday Inn at Salem, having asked for a quiet room facing the river. I think that evening stays in my memory so well because it was the last time he would be close. We had a happy evening with Vint and Maria, and after going out for dinner, spent some time at their house. Dave didn't find it easy to sit still and would wander around, at one time standing in the kitchen as though he didn't know what he was supposed to be doing. We had to keep reminding him to come back and sit down with us, but it was obvious that he sensed the atmosphere of love and acceptance which surounded him.

Maria had volunteered to travel down with us the following day, and I was thankful for this offer. It would be a long and probably exhausting day with a painful good-bye at the end, and her moral support was invaluable.

Our night at the motel passed peacefully. I awoke once and heard geese honking by the riverside, no doubt preparing for their long migration south. It was a comforting sound, with the reassurance that all was well in the realm of nature.

I helped Dave with his bath and dressing the next morning. When bathing him, I noticed how much his body had shrunk, particularly around his shoulders and neck. Also he had trouble standing up and sitting down in the bath, like an old person would. When we were almost ready to leave, I knew I must tell him where we were going. I took my courage in both hands, and told him that we were taking him to the V.A. Hospital at Roseburg. Dr. Masenhimer, who used to be our physician, had moved there, so no doubt he would be seeing him, too. I added this because I felt the familiar name would give him some comfort and indeed he remembered it. He cried a little when I told him this, but offered no opposition. He was completely trusting of whatever decisions I made now. It was hard not to cry myself—he was so pathetically vulnerable and willing to cooperate. I said a prayer of thanks that this hurdle had been overcome and somewhere inside a wordless prayer that he would get through this next experience well; that he would be able to understand we were doing it for the best. How much one longs for comfort for those we love in a situation like this; we cannot reach them often as their understanding is limited, but I have had the feeling that our deepest, unspoken wishes for their needs are perhaps the sincerest prayers we can offer.

We arrived at Vint and Maria's house about 9:30. Vinton was working on his roof, but came down into the house to see us on our way. We joined hands and gathered in a circle for a word of prayer before leaving. I believe that was one of the most emotional prayer times I have ever experienced; there was so much that could only be felt, not spoken, and I felt my own tears rise and overflow. We had been close friends for about seven years, and now one of our number had to be separated from us. How long would it be before the four of us could be together again? What did the future hold? What was the meaning to all of this?

On the drive down we somehow managed to make cheerful conversation, and tried to treat it as another day out to be enjoyed, living in the present, making the most of each moment together. We stopped for lunch at the little town of Sutherlin, ten miles north of Roseburg. I felt anxiety and anticipation creeping through my bones as the time came nearer for this new parting. I know Maria felt the tension too, but Dave, who I think by this time had forgotten where we were going, was the only one who seemed quite relaxed and able to enjoy himself. He even suggested having dinner this evening together, something I just had no answer for. Oh, God, grant that they will be kind and understanding to him in this new setting. Ease the pain of parting somehow; help us to get through this afternoon. As we pulled off at the Roseburg exit, Dave said "This is where we split, isn't it?" Evidently, he did have some recollection of what I had told him. I just nodded; my heart was too full to answer.

It was about one o'clock when we arrived at the admissions desk, but everyone was out to lunch, so we were told to wait for about twenty minutes. As waiting was not one of Dave's strong points, we went out again and walked around the rose garden. The setting of this hospital was magnificent, a large park of about 300 acres with a golf course and many different varieties of trees and shrubs, surrounded by lush, green countryside with tree-covered hills in the background. It is an area still largely unspoiled by industry, and retains much of its natural beauty. The hospital is built of mellow, red brick with white trim. There were about five separate buildings containing the different wards, and houses on the property for some of the staff.

Back at the admissions desk, we announced our presence once more, and the clerk said she would go and check with Mr. House, the admissions director. We sat down and waited for almost an hour; the delay was trying to all of us, to say the least. This was the psychiatric ward, and one of the patients kept walking up and down and looking us over, which didn't make the waiting any easier. He knew we were strange, and finally came up to me, trying to make conversation and shaking my hand. I responded as best I could. Finally, he became rowdy with one of the male aides and was bustled off unceremoniously back to his ward. A nurse arrived and asked Dave to come into the admitting room. We went through the procedure of filling out the tedious forms, having him weighed, and his blood pressure and pulse rate taken. Then back again to the waiting room. Eventually, after about another half-hour, we were ushered into the doctor's office. He was an intelligent-looking oriental gentleman, who once again asked us the same routine questions. He then asked Dave some questions to test his mental ability, and of course quite soon Dave didn't understand and could not answer. He broke down and cried. To me at this point, the pain was excruciating. Both the doctor and I hastened to assure him we were trying to help him.

127

To my horror and amazement, we discovered that there was no written record of the telephone conversation between Mary Lindstrom and Bill House, hence the long delay. This doctor had not been notified of his admission, and asked me if I was going to take him back to the nursing home. The answer was an emphatic no. I went through the whole story once more of the conversation between Mary and Bill, confirming his acceptance here, and the verbal assurance that this would be the admitting day. We had clearance to prove it, but still there was no evidence in writing. The doctor searched his notes for the past few days, then left the room for a while. When he got back the strain became too much for me, and I started to weep myself. He was sympathetic, and finally the tangle was unsnarled; we were escorted upstairs to the third floor, with a male nurse. We had carried his suitcases in with us, but here we were informed that he would not be needing his own clothes for the time being. They would be using ward clothes until they had decided where he would be placed.

Now the time I had dreaded all day had come—the time of leaving him there in those strange surroundings, with strange people, a different environment. I felt like a traitor. A kindly looking young aide came forward and introduced himself, saying he would be taking care of Dave. He advised us to leave as soon as possible. We walked toward the door, and Dave, of course, followed. We turned to say good-bye, and he was restrained from following us. I saw a desperate, bewildered look on his face as the door closed. Oh, supreme agony of that moment. The world is full of pain, deadening, numbing pain, and my own grief began to overflow as we went down in the elevator. Once in the car, I could give full rein to my sorrow. It is like being crucified, having to leave him here, not fully understanding why. Oh God, take care of him—he is so helpless, so utterly at the mercy of those who care for him. May they be kind, understanding, compassionate. It was some time before I could pull myself together, and we were able to start for home. Maria, with infinite patience and understanding, encouraged me to cry, to get it all out. I was profoundly grateful for the fact that she was there. I don't know how I could have coped on the long drive back alone, bearing the pain of this new separation.

The following day was spent mostly in a blur of numbness, going through the motions of life mechanically. I couldn't get my mind away from Dave, and how his first night had been—how was he feeling?

My day was brightened considerably when that afternoon, the social worker called. That morning, two or three of them had spent about an hour with Dave, trying to evaluate him, asking him questions. Some of these questions he could answer, others obviously not, so he needed to verify with me several things which were not clear, and also to get some background on Dave's life.

It was an immense relief to respond to his questions, and also to know that the staff were really interested in his case. I was told that he had cried a lot that morning during the interview, no doubt both because he couldn't answer all their questions and was aware of it, and also because of the new situation, the strangeness. He must have been intensely lonely, lost, and insecure that first day; his feelings of desolation can only be imagined. It was good therapy for me to talk to the social worker, as he allowed me to pour out my feelings about the whole experience; he had been well trained and listened attentively.

He was also able to give me the reason for the long delay in admission. Apparently, Dave's file had been mislaid somewhere on its way from Mr. House's office up to the admitting doctor, but it had been found and all was now well.

About a week later, I became anxious to see him again and could wait no longer. I decided to stay the night at a motel, which would give me an opportunity for two days of visiting. I arrived at Ward 6 about three that afternoon, and asked if I could see him. This was my first experience with a locked ward, which contained psychiatric patients in various stages, most of whom were undergoing rehabilitation. There was a glass partition between the nurses' office and the day room, and someone was on duty at all times in this room. As the nurse left to get him, I looked curiously through the glass, craning my neck to see if he was in sight. After about five minutes, Dave appeared, escorted oy the nurse. He was wearing ward clothes which were much too big for him, but otherwise looked spotlessly clean.

We hugged each other in glad reunion, and I promised I would have him back in time for dinner at five o'clock. We went out into the grounds and walked, talked, and sat for quite a while, just admiring the view and the peaceful surroundings. He seemed quite calm, but had lost some weight, which was not surprising after the shock of this change. There wasn't time that day to go for a drive, but I told them I would be back the next morning to take him out. When I arrived about 9:30, he was already out on a bus ride with some of the other patients—this was a twice-weekly event, to give them a change of scene.

The nurse on duty offered to show me 'round the ward, as most of the patients were out, either on the bus ride or having therapy of different kinds. It was large, spacious, and clean with big windows and immaculately polished floors. Dave's bed was in a big dormitory with about twenty other patients. An exercise ground opened out of the dining room through a glass door. It was completely fenced, and had picnic tables and chairs for those who enjoyed being outside. Here, there was freedom to walk, to be alone, to get away for those who needed to.

While I was waiting for Dave's return, I looked into the front office, and there, much to my joy, was Dr. Masenhimer, getting ready for the day's rounds. It was so good to see him— here was a familiar face, a link with the past. He was most cordial in his welcome and promised he would be visiting Dave within a day or two.

Dave seemed tired during our outing that day. We had lunch at the Windmill Restaurant which was crowded and busy. He had difficulty concentrating and had to be constantly reminded to eat. The new routine on Ward 6 would undoubtedly be full, as this was a rehabilitative ward, but I wondered if perhaps the activities to begin with were too much for him to absorb and he needed more time to adjust.

Perhaps I attempted too much with him that day, since he had already been out for a bus ride that morning. After our lunch, we drove out to Wildlife Safari, only a few miles south of Rose-burg—a big game park covering many acres where the animals had been placed in a natural setting. It was a hot September after-noon, and I don't think he really took in too much, but at least enjoyed being out in the car. It was difficult to get him to focus on the animals for any length of time. The high spot of that tour was having our picture taken holding a four-month-old lion cub called Alex! I am sure I enjoyed this more than he did; he seemed somewhat overwhelmed by it all and not too comfortable.

Not long after this, Carol called and said she was planning to come up for a weekend. This was good news and such a help for me to have her moral support. It made the whole difference, having her to talk to on the long drive, and relieved the weari-ness and monotony. I felt really close to Carol on this visit; we discussed many things—things that were important to us, and we got to know each other that weekend on a much deeper level. I valued her friendship, her warmth, her interest in Dave's and my problem, and her courage in being available and ready to help at a time like this. It was not easy for her to get away, with four children and a husband to take care of, and since they lived in Livermore, California, distance would prevent her from making this trip often.

In fantastic October weather, we drove to Roseburg. I knew she was apprehensive about how she would find him—would she be able to cope? I tried to prepare her as best I could, and we were able to share our apprehension, our fears, our longings for him. It helped so much. When we arrived at the hospital, we paused for a minute in the parking lot and had a word of prayer—prayer for courage, for strength, for whatever may be needed to get us through this day. Once again, we stand at the nurses' sta-tion and look through the glass partition into the ward. He is brought out to greet us looking immaculate. A lump rises in my throat as I watch him and Carol embrace each other. He is not really sure who she is at this moment. Their lives have been sep-arated so much, especially when she was growing up. She had shared with me the fact that he took off frequently, and was an irresponsible father in many ways—immature at that time. Yet she loves him deeply and really cares. This illness has brought us all closer together in a mysterious way—perhaps that is the reason for it?

That Sunday was memorable for many reasons, but most of all because we were all three together as a family. We took him to church that morning—a simple, informal service held in one of the offices on the main floor—and he was able to sit through most of the service, though sometimes would say something unintelligible, evidently trying to join in, though not always at the right moment.

We took a long drive into the country that afternoon. The beauty surrounding us was superb, the trees splashed with gold and burnished copper against a brilliant blue sky, with green, tree-studded hills stretching away in all directions. The countryside around Roseburg is still largely agricultural, and as a result, unspoiled. On one of these country roads, we encountered a house being moved bodily on a flat-bodied truck. We had to wait for some time and then progress was at a snail's pace for several miles, but it brought variety and novelty into our day. The choice of restaurants in the Roseburg area is limited, so we drove north to Sutherlin for lunch, taking the old road which is much more picturesque than the freeway.

We had real problems in getting Dave to sit long enough to finish his lunch. He was up and trying to leave long before the bill was brought. I tried to treat it humorously and asked, "Don't you like our company?" This restlessness was a strange compulsion over which he had no control. I had to ask Carol to hold him while I paid the bill, otherwise he would have walked out of the door and vanished.

We then drove east into more beautiful, rural country along a road which eventually became a mountain trail. At this point we stopped to pick some dried flowers for Carol to take home, and enjoyed basking in the warm sunshine for about half an hour. Then followed the thirty-mile drive back to the hospital at a leisurely pace, wishing that this day didn't have to come to an end, trying to put off taking him back to Ward 6. My heart sank as we arrived once more in the hospital grounds. It seemed so cruel to have to put him back on that locked ward after a time out where his life had been somewhat close to what it used to be before the days of hospitals became necessary. He offered no resistance going back into the building. A nurse greeted us warmly and seemed genuinely interested to hear about our day. Then she told Dave to say good-bye and as Carol hugged him, I saw his face crumple. How well I understand why people often avoid saying good-bye—the wrench, especially in these circumstances, is altogether too much.

I wonder how it seemed to him, going back on the ward, and whether he cried much that evening? How much of our day did he remember? That was the last time we would see him on Ward 6, because the same week he was transferred to the nursing-home unit. Before my next visit, I called to see how he was getting on, and was told he had been transferred. Next time I came down, would I please bring some clothes, as while on Ward 6 he had been using ward clothes almost exclusively, now he would be wearing his own.

I was impressed by the nursing home. It was on the third floor of the main building and ran the whole length of that building. It was tastefully decorated in harmonious colors of light blue and yellow. At the entrance to the day room, there were two canaries in their cages which were looked after by the patients; also an aquarium with many species of brightly colored fish. The room was arranged so that there were small private alcoves where those who didn't want to watch TV could sit and read, or write letters. In addition, there was another TV room adjacent to the dining area.

Dave's room was at the west end of the ward, and again was nicely decorated with light-green walls and attractive curtains; there were four others in the room with him, which was so much nicer than the large dormitory on Ward 6. In addition to clothes, I was asked to bring any photos or albums of his background, so that the nurses would have a better idea of where he came from, his family, and his time in the Marine Corps.

Virginia Grant, the nurse who was assigned to Dave, was most helpful and more than willing to answer any questions I

133

might have. The atmosphere was warm and friendly. Shirley Purcell, the head nurse, was responsible for this congenial atmosphere and had done her best to make the surroundings as close to home as possible. The general impression was one of light and cheerfulness, and the ward was spotlessly clean.

Shirley told me that this ward is a nurse-administered unit, containing mostly patients with chronic illnesses such as Huntington's, Multiple Sclerosis, Alzheimer's Disease, and so on. They do not accept any patients whose life span is likely to be less than three months. There are a total of seventy-five men on the ward, ranging in age from thirty-three to ninety-eight. She and the staff try to make it a place where life can be lived to the fullest; in other words, quality of life is stressed. The men on this ward are referred to as residents, not patients.

Those patients who were well enough, convalescing, and not seriously handicapped, were encouraged to help in different ways, and in a very short time Dave was befriended by two of them, Paul Warner and Arthur Grimberg. They would take him with them down to the dining room for meals—at this time he was still able to eat fairly well by himself, if reminded. Also, they were both garden enthusiasts and would take him out to the rose garden and into the greenhouse when the weather was good. Their kindness and concern for him was touching; Paul even went so far as to ask me one day what foods Dave liked or disliked, so that I could make a list for him.

Virginia told me that when Dave first came on to the nursing-home unit, he was fairly independent. He was still able to dress himself and she would lay out his clothes for him, so that he wouldn't be able to put on two or three sweaters by mistake. Sometimes he needed supervision and often it took him quite a while to get dressed. He was not incontinent either, but they would see to it that he was taken to the bathroom regularly. The only times when he was difficult was when he had to have a shower, have his clothes changed, or be taken to the bathroom. He was helpful, and would often assist cleaning up after meals, stacking the trays, wiping down the trolleys, and so forth. His speech at that time was still quite good, but his answers were sometimes out of context, off the point, or not related to the question. Sometimes he could shave himself, but often his mind would wander and he would not finish. He would walk up and down a lot on the ward; sometimes running when he got agitated, but as much as possible he was free to be himself, within certain limits. Toward the end of his time at Roseburg, he had to be poseyed* in bed at night until he went to sleep, otherwise he would get up and start pacing. This was not a locked ward; the elevator opened directly on to the floor, so on several occasions, he walked into it and went down or up as the case might be, ending up on another floor.

There were seventy-five patients on this ward, and three of them had Alzheimer's Disease; Dave made the fourth.

Quite often on our drives now, he would fall asleep. The car always had a soothing effect on him. He paced so much on the ward that when in the car, he would relax and fall asleep. It was probably needed, but it meant that he never saw some of the lovely country we drove through. It may be that by this time, scenery didn't mean much anymore as he was unable to focus. Sometimes, there were problems when I took him to a restaurant alone. One day we drove about thirty miles east of the hospital to have lunch at a restaurant that had been recommended by one of the nurses. It was quite busy when we got there, and we had to wait some time to be served. Dave started to fidget with his knife and fork and placemat. Eventually I had to tell him to stop as it was getting on my nerves. Instead of being irritated, he laughed, and didn't seem to mind at all being corrected. We had an excellent lunch, but I knew that afterwards I was going to have to go to the ladies' room and with no one to supervise Dave, I didn't know how I could manage it. So I saw him safely into the men's room, told him to wait for me and then dashed into the ladies'. I was not quick enough, however, as when I came out he had vanished completely. I looked up and

---

*Poseyed—a soft waist restraint (Posey belt) applied to prevent falling or getting up without assistance, but which still allows some movement.

down, then went back into the dining room but he was nowhere to be seen. I asked two of the waitresses if they had seen him, but with no result. I had horrible visions of him wandering out on to the road and being hit by a car, or getting lost completely somewhere in the woods. Once more, I went back into the passage by the kitchen and out of the back door. To my profound relief, Dave appeared as mysteriously as he had vanished, walking toward me from the back yard of the restaurant. He must have wandered out quite a long way, then, fortunately realizing he was on strange ground, turned and came back. My knees were weak with suspense, and I gratefully hurried him into the car for our drive back. At this stage, and in fact for some time previously, he no longer recognized our car and would often try to get into the wrong car when we came out from a restaurant.

Toward the end of October, I heard that there was a possibility he might be transferred to the V.A. Hospital at Tacoma. They had a research ward there for Alzheimer patients, and were looking for someone who was still in good physical condition. They had contacted Roseburg to see if there was anyone suitable, and Dave's name had been given. The other Alzheimer patients at the nursing home were apparently not in good enough physical condition to be considered. It came as a shock to me that we might have to face another move so soon after he had come to Roseburg. To be honest, I hoped that it wouldn't happen, and since the details had not yet been worked out, I pushed it into the back of my mind, hoping it wouldn't come to pass.

During November, he came down with a urinary-tract infection which left him very weak. Virginia told me that he had run a fever for a couple of days, so she put him to bed and got the doctor immediately. He was over the worst of it when I came down for Thanksgiving, but still looked very pale and had lost quite a bit of weight. The day before Thanksgiving I took him out to dinner; it was the first time he had been off the ward for about two weeks. He looked so awfully pale that I hesitated, thinking perhaps I was running a risk taking him out in his weakened state. But the nurses encouraged me to go ahead—they thought a change of scene would be good for him. We went to a Chinese restaurant and it was almost impossible to get him to concentrate on his food. His mind wandered constantly, and he stared around the room, distracted by the other people and all the talk and noise. His appearance was beginning to change drastically now, and he had a gaunt, haggard look. Also his expression was different, I suppose because he no longer focused normally.

The next day was Thanksgiving, and Shirley had kindly offered to let us have lunch on the ward together with a private table to ourselves. It was to be at about one o'clock, and Dr. Masenhimer and his wife had said they would come up and see us while we were eating as he was the medical doctor on call. It was a gray, still morning with no wind, and after our morning drive, we came back to the ward and sat together in a small lounge near his room. I hoped so much to be able to talk to him for a while—that he would be able to sit quietly without pacing, just so that we could be together. It would mean so very much if he could do this. While we were sitting there, one of the questions he asked was, "Where do I go from here?" I felt completely inadequate to answer in any way, this question was so unexpected. I said, "Do you know the Lord is with you?" holding his hand tightly.

He seems to register, and says, "Yes, I know." Soon after, he wanders off again and leaves me sitting alone, reading. There doesn't seem to be anything else to do, as I don't feel like walking up and down the ward with him. A wave of loneliness, dejection, desolation sweeps over me. Oh God, my heart is exceedingly sorrowful. I suppose this is the beginning of harder times yet to come, and once again I make the mistake of looking down the dark avenues of the future. But the question is, how much worse can it get before he finally leaves this world? I fear what other roads I may be led down before this is finished. I pray to you, as I have so often in the past, to have mercy. I believe it is my heart's desire that you should take him from this life soon, but you understand that this is something I may ask in ignorance, and I can only trust you to answer according to your infinite wisdom and knowledge of the whole situation. You gave us our lives and they are yours to take back as it pleases you. Our timing is never the same as yours.

I was jolted out of my reverie by a nurse who asked me if I had seen Dave lately. I had assumed that he was still pacing up and down the ward, but apparently he had gone down in the elevator. A search party is alerted, and I go down myself to the first floor to see if I can find him. I learned from the receptionist that someone had already been sent outside to look, and the V.A. police had also been notified. After about twenty minutes, he was found, in the south parking lot, which strangely enough, is where my car was parked. I wonder if he had some idea that I was still out there, and that perhaps he would find me?

When we sat down for our Thanksgiving dinner, he looked exhausted and was still somewhat restless. He would pick up his fork and take a mouthful or two, then put it down and stare around him. I kept encouraging him to eat, but he didn't seem to have much appetite. The food was superb: roast turkey, sage and herb stuffing, mashed potatoes, fresh vegetables, a delicious salad, and rolls. The dietician had put on an outstanding meal and it seemed such a shame that he was not able to really enjoy it.

Dr. Masenhimer and his wife, Gladys, came on to the ward and sat with us while we were eating. That made it even harder for Dave to concentrate, as of course they were talking to him. I was so grateful for their kindness in coming to be with us—it was good to feel their support and understanding. Dave was obviously pleased to see them; he remembered the doctor quite well and had always thought a lot of him. For me, conversation was difficult because of my preoccupation with Dave and his food; how I wished he could enjoy this time as we would have in normal circumstances; nevertheless, it is the closest we can get to normal, things being what they are.

December 3, 1978. It is Dave's birthday and Kathy Jones, who so kindly befriended us while he was at the nursing home, has offered to come down with me and stay overnight so that we can be there with him to celebrate. So once more I have a companion on the long four-hour drive. We arrive Saturday afternoon and go up to the ward for a visit. Dave seems to recognize her, or at least is aware that she is someone who he once knew. Kathy has always had a flair for dealing with patients (I noticed this at the nursing home). She has real compassion and is able to listen genuinely and enter into their conversation.

His birthday fell on a Sunday that year, so in the morning, we took him to church. He grew restless, sometimes talked at the wrong moment, or fidgeted, and I knew that the times when I would be able to take him to church were now limited. Our drive afterwards took us to Denny's for coffee and refreshments, Kathy managing to keep him in conversation and he responding quite well for a while. She seems to be able to get through to him, or is it that because even now he is able to put up a better front with someone he doesn't know so well?

The birthday party was shared with one of the other patients, and the staff really put themselves out to make it a special day for both of them. Each one had his own individual cake with icing and a candle. Everyone gathered 'round and sang "Happy Birthday to You." Dave couldn't take in what was happening; his attention was distracted and he found it hard to eat. As soon as he could, he got up and wandered off to continue pacing up and down as usual.

Usually, I stayed on the ward until well into the afternoon before driving back, but today Kathy wanted to get home to have some time with her mother before going to work the next day. She worked full time as a hostess-cashier in a restaurant, so had given up her weekend to come down and see Dave with me. As we left, he was being taken out for a Sunday-afternoon bus ride; I remember him waving to us as he left, escorted by a nurse. He seemed quite content and not at all disturbed that we were leaving.

About ten days before Christmas, I flew down to Roseburg for the day. The plane was delayed due to fog and I didn't arrive until just about lunchtime. I called the hospital asking them if they could hold his lunch so I could take him out, but he had already started his meal. I also learned that the date for his transfer to the V.A. Hospital at Tacoma, had been set for January 9, so he only had about three weeks left here.

He was in good spirits that day, I remember, and looked much better having now recovered from the effects of his bladder infection. We went for a long drive that afternoon, stopping at a gift shop where I bought him a china English setter for Christmas. In the shop, he didn't seem to focus at all, just stared straight ahead of him and seemed anxious to leave. Once back in the car, he was in good spirits again and we took a long drive out into the country east of Roseburg. It rained heavily all the way, but Dave didn't seem depressed at all and talked to me quite a bit that day. It was one of those rare times when I felt he really was aware of what was going on, so I made the most of it. As mentioned before, the motion of the car seemed to soothe him, but today he noticed quite a few things—remarked when he saw a dog or other animal on the road and waved to some passersby when we were going slowly through a town.

After our drive, I stayed on the ward until about 4:30, then Dr. Masenhimer came up and I drove back to their house for dinner. It was a delightful evening, with their three boys also at home. His wife, Gladys, is a warm, wonderful person with a great sense of humor, and it was a joy to spend that evening with such a happy, united family.

I knew now that I would only have one more visit to Roseburg and that would be for Christmas, when I had planned to go down for two nights. So this phase of our lives was also coming to an end. I felt sad, somewhat nostalgic. It had been only four months, and after the strain and trauma of leaving him there, it seemed too soon for another change. He was really settled in on the nursing home, had good care, perhaps as good as I could hope for, so I had very mixed feelings about this transfer.

When talking to Vinton earlier about the proposed change, he said that of course, if I wished, I could refuse and just leave him at Roseburg, but he felt that we should try as much as possible to go along with what the hospital suggested, believing it was in Dave's best interests. I admit that I was not wholehearted about the change, even though it had been pointed out that he would get more attention on this research ward. There were only fifteen patients, all Alzheimer's, as against seventy-five on the Roseburg ward. Also, I was told that there was a wives' group at Tacoma, which met once a month for mutual support, so on the face of it, it seemed that this move must be for the best.

Dr. Masenheimer had said I could use their house when I went down to visit at Christmas. They would be away, but would be glad to have someone staying there and gave me a key. I took Dave for a long walk in the grounds that afternoon of December 23, the day I arrived. It was wet and muddy from recent heavy rains, and when we got back to the hospital, I took his boots off to clean them. I discovered that his feet were badly blistered from all the pacing up and down, plus this long walk. An aide at once came to the rescue and suggested we soak his feet and put some ointment on. I knew now that the boots were too heavy and no longer fitted properly, thus causing these blisters. His feet had probably shrunk and changed shape as the disease progressed. Also, I was told later that these patients change their walk as time goes on, putting the weight on a different part of the foot. He enjoyed having his feet soaked and sat quietly while we did it.

Christmas morning dawned cold and dry and I took him out for a ten-mile drive before coming back in for lunch. Once again we were going to have our own table on the ward, and this time it would be shared with another patient and his wife, who was also down for Christmas. As at Thanksgiving, the meal was superb and the table gaily decorated with Christmas greens and a red tablecloth. Dave managed fairly well and ate a bit more this time, but any conversation distracted him and it was a job to make him sit still long enough to finish. The nurses were especially kind and attentive that day. After lunch came the opening of presents which was a big event. Every patient on the ward had a gift to be opened and it was a time of great excitement. Dave was thoroughly confused since the whole thing meant nothing to him. He was anxious to get away from all the noise and turmoil. Strange, he had always been that way at family gatherings at his mother's house. When everyone else was celebrating, he would go upstairs to get away by himself. The gift opening took some time, which was natural—why shouldn't these men make the most of Christmas and the kindness which had been extended to them? For Dave, however, it was just more confusion. I tried to keep him with me and help him to join in, but eventually, he became quite angry and irritable, so I let him go and he started pacing again, though at the other end of the ward, as far away as possible from the festivities.

Before leaving that afternoon, I took a short walk around the parking lot. I had come to feel at home here, but this was to be the last time for us at Roseburg. In just two weeks from now, I would be back again to take him on the long journey north, for I had agreed to be his escort on the plane to Seattle. Shirley had told me that transport would be arranged to the Eugene airport on the morning of January 9, probably about 10:30, which would give us ample time to catch our plane at 1:15. I looked 'round the now-familiar grounds which I had come to know well during the last four months, and felt real regret that this had to be the end of our sojourn here. As I started home a bitter north wind was blowing which was to herald the beginning of an icy spell for the next two weeks. Once home again, I braced myself for the move which was to come. This would be the third major change for us within a year.

The week of January 7 started off with icy frozen ground. So far, we had had no snow, but heavy frost each night for the past ten days. A warming trend was predicted, much to my relief, as it was due to come just in time for my journey down to Roseburg. I had a plane reservation for the morning of the eighth, but well before daylight I awoke to the sound of cracking branches, crashing trees, and flashes of blue flame, as one by one, the power lines went down. We were in the midst of an ice storm, which paralyzed all movement that day. A two-inch coating of ice covered everything: roads, trees, roofs, shrubs—the scene was one of devastation. There was no electricity in the house, and for the time being life had come to a standstill. Fortunately, the phone was still working, so I called the hospital to tell them it was impossible for me to get down that day. They had already heard the news of the weather conditions, so it was agreed that Dave's move would be cancelled till the next day. The airport was closed, and driving on those icy roads was out of the question. By midday, things had improved slightly and the Greyhound buses were running, so I decided to take the next one out, which would get me into Roseburg at about 8:30 that evening.

I left the house somewhat reluctantly, as the power was still off and there was no heat or light. I had a hot meal before boarding the bus and put my car in a garage in downtown Portland. As it turned out, that bus ride was a chance to get some rest after the trauma of the ice storm and my preparations for Dave's journey. I slept most of the way down, too tired even to think about tomorrow and what it might bring.

When we arrived in Roseburg it was raining hard, and was quite mild, which seemed a good omen for our journey, if these conditions held up. I walked from the bus station to a nearby motel and checked in thankfully for the night. It occurred to me that perhaps I should call the hospital to find out if tomorrow's plans were still the same, but I was so tired that the thought of having to battle with any more details was too much. Let tomorrow take care of itself. I slept well and woke early, contacting the ward about seven o'clock.

The plans had been changed. Instead of having a car to Eugene airport leaving about 10:30, now we were to go in the hospital van, which left at 8:30, thereby giving us at least a three-and-a-half-hour wait for our plane. I ate a hurried breakfast and took a taxi over to the hospital. Dave greeted me with a big hug; he was dressed and all ready to go, but we were told we had to hurry in order to be ready in time, and his packing was not yet finished. Hastily, Virginia and I packed the remaining clothes in his room; there were still some in the laundry which would have to be sent on later.

I felt upset that our departure from that ward had to be so frenzied; I was also angry that the plans had been changed at the last minute without any notice. There was no time to say goodbye to the other staff as we hurried downstairs to the travel agent's office to pick up our tickets. It so happened that Dr. Masenhimer was down there at the same time, so we did have a minute for a brief exchange with him. He greeted us both warmly and wished us a good trip. Dave was so cooperative, completely trusting, quite happy to be with me and to do whatever I said. He was aware he was going on an outing, but I am sure could not have understood what it was all about.

Virginia took us out the back door to where the bus was waiting. We said our final good-byes, and then we were on our way. It was about 8:45, and with a sinking heart I wondered how on earth we were going to get through this long wait. I felt real sorrow at our departure from Roseburg; the care at the nursing home had been outstanding, such a relief to me to know he was well and compassionately cared for. Now we had to face another change, adjust to a new setting, more strange people. It was like starting all over again.

The drive to Eugene went smoothly. Dave always enjoyed the car, and was quite content and relaxed. There were several other patients in the van with us, and we chatted back and forth from time to time. It was just ten o'clock as we drew into the Eugene airport. Our last link with Roseburg had come to an end, and it was with a feeling of distinct apprehension that we bade the driver good-bye and walked into the crowded airport. Now we were really on our own, and there was no one I knew to turn to for help, if it should be needed. I felt very much alone at that moment. We checked in at the ticket counter and I explained that he was a V.A. patient and I was traveling as his escort. Almost the first thing I asked the attendant to do was take him to the men's room. They were extremely busy that day, but he rose splendidly to the occasion and took Dave at once. What a relief—at least that was behind us for the time being!

The first hour wasn't too bad. He seemed to be quite interested watching the people come and go. There was a lot of activity with most people waiting for delayed flights to arrive— flights that had been cancelled the day before. How thankful I was that we hadn't attempted this journey yesterday.

Sometimes we walked up and down inside to pass the time, then would go outside for a while to get away from the crowd. Mercifully, it wasn't raining. Because his boots were too big and heavy to pack, I had to carry them in one hand and hold on to him with the other. He was wearing comfortable leather slippers which were much better for his feet. People were obviously noticing the way he looked and that I had to hold on to him constantly. I saw their curious stares and knew that they were talking about us. I felt so sick of being hemmed in by people who don't understand. How could they? I don't give a damn what they think. I love him—he is my husband. I made a phone call to Vinton, hoping against hope that he might be free and able to come down and spend some time with us, as it's only about an hour's drive from his house, but there was no answer. Anything, anything to pass the time. Now he was beginning to get agitated, impatient, not understanding this laborious wait. At 11:30 or thereabouts, we went and had lunch. The service was slow, but it didn't matter. I tried to make him focus on the airfield, to watch what was going on out there, but as usual, he was distracted by the crowds of milling people in the restaurant. He ate a fairly good lunch, however, and at least that passed almost another hour for us. We learned that flight 773 to Seattle would be late arriving—it would not now be in till 1:45.

Dave is restless: "Let's go, let's go," he kept saying. I don't know how many times I had to explain the reason for our wait—I must have sounded like a stuck record. I felt desperation growing. The awful thought came to me that perhaps the plane would be cancelled altogether. What then? I would have to find a motel for us in Eugene overnight. I am on the point of breaking down as we walk and walk and walk. I apologized to Dave for being short, snapping at him. It is amazing how good he is, all things considered, but I had to stay with him all the time. It would not be safe to leave him sitting alone, even for a few minutes. It's like being in a trap—we can't get away from these people who are waiting, waiting, waiting, endlessly waiting. Oh God, how bad I am at waiting—how futile seem the things we do to pass the time. How much of life is spent waiting, waiting, waiting. It must have a purpose, I suppose.

Finally, just before 2:00 P.M., the plane arrived; we had been at the airport four hours. We crowded into the departure lounge and once more we had to sit and wait while the passengers came off; ten minutes, fifteen minutes; desperation builds again. Surrounded and hemmed in by people, we can hardly move and Dave starts to get tense and mutter to himself, tugging at my hand

and trying to back away. When the announcement comes to board, it is almost unbelievable. Once we were in our seats, things seemed better, but I noticed that the fog was closing in and unless we could get off the ground pretty soon, perhaps we wouldn't leave at all. I went through another twenty minutes of desperation before we taxied out to take off.

At last the tension was eased. The flight to Seattle was smooth and beautiful. It made all those hours of waiting seem as nothing. Mt. St. Helens and Mt. Rainier stick their snow-capped peaks out of swirling clouds, providing us with a magnificent view of their volcanic cones. It is a different world up here and at least we are moving now to our destination.

We arrived in Seattle and walked down to the baggage-claim area. The driver from the V.A. Hospital was there to meet us and we watched as the first load of baggage came down the ramp. Once more, we sit and wait, sit and wait, sit and wait. The driver from the hospital was helpful, patient. He must have been through experiences like this many times. He showed no signs of irritation. I felt again on the point of a breakdown. How could this happen to us just when we needed so much to be on our way? Anything to have this journey finished. Will we ever get out of here?

The driver, noticing that I was on the verge of tears, suggested that we leave without the baggage, but I could not bear another complication—there are important papers in that suitcase—records he would need for admission. We waited a full hour, then finally the baggage came off and we were on our way to the car and the last stage of our journey.

How vulnerable I am to the minor frustrations of life. How I resent having to suffer this kind of trial. In the car on the way to the hospital I looked at Dave and thought, *What an example he is to me!* His features were relaxed; he seemed to be entering into and enjoying the variety of experiences he had been through today. Above all, I marvel at his complete trust in me; his unquestioning obedience and cooperation to go wherever I suggest, to do what he is asked. I wonder how it feels to be without defenses, as he is most of the time now. Once again, I wish so much I could enter his world if only for a few moments, just to understand how that world feels, how things appear to him.

Dave, I love you so much. Perhaps never before have you been so lovable, for now you are completely open, living for the moment. I don't think the past or the future have any reality for you—just the "now." Therefore you're not anxious what may happen. What can I learn from this?

8.   Walking the Precipice at Tacoma

The drive from the Seattle airport to the V.A. Hospital at Tacoma is about forty miles. Darkness was falling as we drove in at the hospital gates and down a long avenue to the admissions building. The drive was lined with tall firs and a row of Norwegian silver maples. Our driver escorted us in to the admissions office, which was quiet at this time of day, the regular work hours having finished for most of the staff. I handed in Dave's medical records and the admissions clerk then asked him a few general questions: his name and his parents' names, both of which he was able to answer.

We sat and waited awhile before a psychiatrist appeared— he had been called at home to come back and do the admitting procedure before Dave could be taken on to the ward. He asked several questions to test his awareness and sense of reality, but this interview was not in any way as traumatic as the one we had experienced at Roseburg. It took less than half an hour, and the doctor then contacted the ward and asked them to send some- one over to escort us there. A young male aide appeared shortly, and drove us to Ward 85B. It must have been about six when we finally got there, and I knew Dave must be hungry, as we had eaten lunch early while waiting for our plane at Eugene. The first thing I did was to ask the nurse in charge to bring him some food, and before too long a tasty spaghetti dinner was served; she also brought a glass of milk for me. Then followed the un- packing of his suitcase and I helped put away his clothes. He was in a room with five or six other patients. I suppose because I was so tired by then, the parting when I finally left the ward was not really painful. Dave seemed quite calm and was walking up and down inspecting his new surroundings.

I took a taxi to a motel, and had dinner about eight P.M. There had been so much to occupy my thoughts that I had not realized how hungry I was. Sleep did not come easily that night, as I was so wound up from our marathon that day. We had been traveling from about 8:30 that morning until after five in the evening—a day of enormous strain with the exhausting waits and accompanying frustration; a day of trying to be patient with Dave, who didn't understand the delays. When I looked back, I wondered how I had been able to survive it at all—my strength was sapped and I knew I had not been able to respond as I would want to. My own impatience at the frustrations we had experienced had drained me to the utmost.

The next morning, the psychiatrist in charge of the ward, Dr. Zem, called me and asked if I could come over to the ward to talk to him. I said I had no car this time so we did it over the phone. He went extensively into Dave's life and background with me, covering not only the routine events of his life, but his personality traits and general tendencies when he was still normal. It gave me a chance to ask him many questions that were on my mind too, and once again it was good therapy to pour out some of my feelings.

I had a plane reservation back to Portland that day, and soon after my conversation with the doctor, took the airport bus back to Seattle. While waiting in line at the ticket counter, I was appalled to learn that the Portland airport was closed due to fog, and would be opened again only if conditions improved. The ticket clerk told me that if there were enough passengers to justify it, they would run a bus to Portland instead. I went and had some lunch, then came back to check again and see if the bus would be running. He expected it would be there within the next fifteen minutes, so once more I sat and waited. A bus appeared and drew up outside the entrance, but no announcement was made, and the driver got out and stood for a while as though

149

waiting to be told how many passengers to expect. I felt my own impatience and resentment rising once more. How could life be so cruel as to hand me another day of waiting after all we had been through yesterday? It seemed so unfair, so unbelievable. I went up and asked the driver if this was the bus for Portland, and he told me he didn't know—he had not yet been informed. I returned to the ticket counter and vented all my pent-up frustration and fury on the ticket clerk. He now said that he wasn't sure if there would be a bus to Portland after all; he didn't think there were enough passengers to make it worthwhile. To say I was hopping mad would be a gross understatement—by this time I was boiling with rage, and after some searing comments to the clerk about lack of consideration for passengers in these circumstances, I promptly went down to the car-rental office. I had taken enough; I just didn't have any reserves of patience, tolerance, or strength left to endure another day of waiting or uncertainty. I knew this was an expensive alternative, but I had to get out of that airport somehow.

Fortunately, there was a car available at the rental office, and thankfully I took it and started the 160-mile drive back to Portland. If I had been calm enough to reason logically, I could have asked one of the other passengers on that cancelled flight to share the rental car with me, thereby reducing the expense, but all I could think of was escape, freedom from any more waiting, no matter what the cost. That airport had become an enemy to me; it was associated with all the pain of waiting, parting, sadness, endurance, uncertainty—all the things that had been such a trial the day before.

The drive back was uneventful, though tiring, because of my own state of mind. I sincerely hoped that the effects of the ice storm would be over when I arrived, but as I entered north Portland, there was still some ice on the trees although it had thawed out on the roads. Gratefully, I drove into the Avis garage to return my car and pick up my own car for the drive home.

A big branch had broken off a Douglas fir at the entrance to our driveway, but otherwise there was no major damage. I was sure that by now, there would be electricity in the house, but to my dismay as I walked in, a cold dark house greeted me. The light switches were still dead, the furnace was still off. What a welcome after two days of intense emotional strain! I was too tired to fight any more, but contacted Delores, my neighbor, who told me that it was expected the power would be restored either tonight or tomorrow morning. Mercifully, the telephone was still working, so I called Gwen and asked if I could come over for the night. The prospect of spending a night in this unheated house alone after all I'd been through was something I couldn't face.

Once again, it came to me how very vulnerable we are to lack of heat, fatigue, and the effects of emotional drain. I dragged myself over to Gwen's house to be greeted with a blazing fire, dinner cooking, a hot bath, a warm bed. Once again, her house was a sanctuary to me in a time of desperate need. Gwen and Cliff were having friends over for dinner, which I remember was an excellent meal. How wonderful finally to be able to relax completely, not to have to struggle any more, or face more problems. That night I slept the sleep of sheer exhaustion.

The next few days were a time of recovery—I was limp and exhausted and just lived automatically without too many feelings of any kind. I sensed a kind of resignation to this new move; there was not the intense pain that had been there after his move to Roseburg. I was gradually being conditioned to learn what it meant to release him in a new and different way. I felt ashamed at my behavior when frustrated at the airport, but perhaps I learned something from it—that I am not superhuman in any way, just as subject to failure and weakness as anyone else.

With the beginning of this phase of our lives at Tacoma, the story inevitably becomes more mine than Dave's. I can only describe his behavior as I saw it during visits to the ward; for obvious reasons I cannot be a daily part of his life now, and after the time at Roseburg I am beginning to realize what this means and gradually to accept it. I decided that I would still visit every ten days, as I had at Roseburg. One consolation was that the drive was somewhat shorter— about twenty miles or so. Accordingly, about ten days after his admission, I went up to see him. He appeared to have settled in reasonably well, but was

151

quite restless, pacing up and down the ward and sometimes running. There was to be an unexpected bonus on that first visit, as while I was talking to one of the nurses, a smiling, gray-haired lady came up and introduced herself. This was Louise, whose husband was also on the same ward. She at once invited me to come and stay with her for the two nights I would be there, and I appreciated this offer of hospitality which was so spontaneous, so unexpected. Even though I had Star with me, that did not seem to upset her in the least, and she was kind enough to tolerate both me and my dog in her apartment!

Louise worked as a volunteer on the ward four or five days a week; together the wives had purchased a washer and dryer to use for clothes which would otherwise have been ruined by the hospital laundry, and it was a familiar sight to see Louise presiding over the washer and dryer in the small laundry room; usually her husband, Bill, would be in there with her. Dave was still able to go out for lunch, so Louise and I took him to the Black Angus steakhouse. He managed quite well with our supervision and encouragement, had a juicy, tender steak and a large dish of ice cream for dessert. Nevertheless, from his behavior that day, I knew the time was very close when he would no longer be able to handle a meal in a restaurant. If he had to wait any length of time, he became fidgety, causing embarrassment to me and the other customers. His gestures and actions were becoming more unpredictable and he needed to be watched carefully all the time.

There were about fifteen other patients on the ward at the time Dave was admitted, all in varying stages of decline. Although most had been diagnosed as having Alzheimer's Disease, the diagnosis by EMI or CAT scan is rarely 100 percent accurate, and only studies of brain tissue removed at autopsy can provide the final answer. The range of decline in these patients was wide—from complete immobility and inability to help themselves up to those similar to Dave, who could still walk, talk to some extent, and feed themselves. In the final stages, the patient becomes completely rigid, totally incontinent, and can only take liquid food, as the muscles controlling swallowing and digestion are affected.

To begin with, those patients in the final stages were really a trial to me, particularly those who were noisy and hostile, also incontinent. Usually, there were puddles of urine on the floor which had to be constantly mopped up, and clothes to be changed perhaps several times a day in some cases. This type of nursing is definitely not "in the book" and requires special training in learning to perceive the needs of a patient who can no longer express himself. Dave at this point was still not incontinent, and would quite often take himself to the bathroom and manage adequately without help if reminded why he was there.

Toward the end of February, Carol again flew up, this time bringing her third daughter, Sherry, who was five years old. She was a real tonic to the ward, like a breath of fresh air, and those patients who were still aware enough to appreciate her were given a special treat by this happy, spontaneous child who solemnly paced up and down the ward, holding her grandpa's hand, running when he ran, completely accepting this situation and not aware of anything unusual about it.

That weekend, we took him out for lunch for what was to be the last time. We drove to MacDonalds for a hamburger, and I can remember clearly Dave sitting hand in hand with Sherry at the table, waiting while Carol and I ordered the hamburgers. His expression of sheer delight as he looked down at his granddaughter will stay in my memory always.

On the day they were due to fly back home, Carol was not feeling well and shortly afterwards came down with the flu; nevertheless she and Sherry came on to the ward that morning for a final visit, and I can only admire her courage and determination in facing the trauma and depression surrounding her and not being overcome by it.

A word now about the research program on this ward. It is entitled the GRECC Program (Geriatric Research Education and Clinical Center). Seven other V.A. hospitals in the country are doing studies on various aspects of aging, but this program is the only one of its kind. It is administered through the Seattle and American Lake V.A. hospitals under the direction of Dr. Murray Raskind. Various studies have been undertaken and are still continuing. These include a sleep study in which an electroencephalogram (EEG) is monitored during both sleep and waking hours to determine how the brain waves of these patients differ from those of normal elderly people, and a study of samples of both blood and spinal fluid which are being analyzed for clues as to abnormalities which might lead ultimately to discovery of the cause of this disease. Another angle of research is the possible dysfunction of the auto-immune system; also neuro-pathological studies covering structural and chemical changes in brain tissue.

During those first months, they were experimenting with different kinds of drugs to calm Dave down and reduce his hectic pacing. To begin with, they tried to do without any medication, but he was so difficult to handle when he had to be showered, shaved, dressed, and so forth, that some degree of medication was essential. He had now reached the stage where often he would not understand what was wanted. It was almost impossible to get through to him verbally, and when having his clothes changed or any other of the necessary functions which had to be done, he would resist, push the nurse away, or be verbally abusive. The object was to discover which drugs would be best suited to him at this particular phase and then to give him a minimum dosage—just enough to relax him without making him dopey. One of the first drugs tried was Lithium, which had mixed results. Although he remained alert, it did not seem to reduce his tension enough to be really effective, and as I remember, his comprehension, limited though it was, became even worse.

I can remember trying to help him with dinner one evening. Louise was feeding one of the bedridden patients, so I took his tray in to that room to be with her. I couldn't get him to sit down to eat, so he took snatches of food standing up or walking around, and if I tried to hold him, kept trying to pull away. He grabbed my hand and squeezed hard until it hurt, and the more I tried to persuade him to eat, the less he seemed to comprehend.

We had a really nice spell of weather during March of that year, so one day I decided to take him out for a picnic lunch. As usual, he was quite peaceful when in the car, but as soon as we got out, he wanted to walk off and had absolutely no idea that he should be sitting down to eat his food. Consequently, I had to again hold him with one hand while feeding him his sandwich with the other. By now any strange place out of doors was beginning to be unfamiliar to him, so he may have felt lost and afraid, or not understood why we were there. As mentioned earlier, it now dawned on me that often these kinds of outings were more for my benefit than for his; since he couldn't now tell me what things he enjoyed, I could only try to do what I thought might be best for him. At this point in time, we were very close to losing verbal communication. Although his speech was fairly good in that he could articulate words and sentences, his understanding and response to questions was often totally out of context.

Shortly afterwards, I first met Harriet, whose husband, Les, was on the same ward. I had been up for my usual two-day visit and was just about to start for home when an attractive lady drove in and parked her car. I was walking Star at the time; she stopped to admire him and said, "What a cute little dog." She introduced herself and we had some conversation before I left. Like Louise, she was destined to become a close friend, so once more, I had been provided with help and support along the way. There were other wives too, walking the same tragic road with their husbands, but Louise and Harriet were the ones I came to know the best. Both had started out earlier on this ward than I, some two years or so, and each in her own way had learned to come to terms with the situation, and in sharing our tragic experiences we found comfort and therapy.

Both Bill and Les shared a two-bed room on the ward, and from the first had taken a liking to each other. And so, I gradually began to adjust to this change and to learn from these two good friends how to handle my visits on the ward. This was not done so much by words as by example. They coped courageously with the pain and frustrations that are inevitable in a separation of this kind. Up until now, I had had to make this journey alone, but now there were two other people who understood, who accepted me, and who had extended a hand of friendship. The bond that comes through mutual suffering of this kind is very special; there is an unspoken understanding, and we sense each other's

155

moods and reactions without having to go into explanations.

Easter, 1979 was a sad time for me. I went up as usual for two days, and the Saturday before Easter, I awoke feeling depressed and weighed down. I think I remembered other, happier Easters, and particularly the year before when he was in the nursing home and had been able to go to the sunrise service with Worth and Elsa. Now it was out of the question to get him to sit long enough through a church service. It was another of the many times when Dave's hopeless future hit me hard; I was talking to Louise in her apartment and suddenly broke down. But tears are therapy, too, and a release from the crushing weight of this burden. Louise accepted my tears and grief as someone who could identify in every way with what I was feeling. Later that day, as I said good-bye to Dave and to these two friends on the ward, they were just leaving to take Bill and Les over to Harriet's house for the afternoon. Dave again was tense and pacing hard—he knew me but was so agitated he could hardly stop or sit down for any length of time.

Tears fell again during the drive home, I remember. I wonder how long this journey will go on? How will I ever find the strength to keep up these visits every ten days?

Later that spring and well into the summer months, there was an acute gas shortage and driving became precarious because the shortage was particularly bad around Tacoma. There were often long lines at most of the gas stations and some were open only two or three hours a day.

Toward the end of May, Louise, Harriet, and I went on a picnic with our three husbands. The hospital is situated close to a huge lake with fishing docks at various points, and there was one especially attractive spot just a short drive from the ward. Harriet took Les in her car; Louise and Bill came with me and Dave. There was some confusion as we started out, as my car was parked close to some bushes, not allowing Dave enough room to get in on the passenger's side. I let him in on the driver's side, hoping to move him over to the other seat. As anyone who has dealt with an Alzheimer patient will know, it is extremely difficult to redirect them, get them to understand directions or change

156

course. He sat happily behind the wheel, convinced he was going to drive! After much maneuvering, I managed to pry him loose from the driver's seat, and asked Harriet to hold him while I moved the car out so he could get in on the passenger's side. Anyone observing us during these moments would have been treated to a first-class comedy show! We ourselves collapsed into giggles because the whole operation seemed so ludicrous. After arriving at the lake side, we unpacked our lunch. I had brought two cartons of Seven-up in a paper bag. I had to hold on to Dave in case he walked off, so had him in one hand and my Seven-up in the other. The bag had become soggy and burst, spilling its contents on the ground and all over Dave's feet. "Oh . . ." he said. At least he was aware enough to know that something was wrong! I was left holding aloft a sodden, empty paper bag in my other hand.

This was probably the beginning of the time when I learned how to laugh at the small, everyday things that happened, and to see humor on days when I would have thought it was impossible. What a lifesaver is the gift of laughter. I was to discover that it can be found even in the darkest places.

Our picnic went off well and Dave managed to stand still long enough to eat. He walked with me out on to the dock, looked down at the water, and said, "Have you brought your fishing poles?" After lunch, there was no holding him, so I had perforce to leave and walk with him, leaving Louise and Harriet, Bill and Les to socialize together. Days such as this are a major triumph—it was a lovely picnic in which our husbands were able to join. All three were having a "good" day, and really seemed to know they were on an outing.

On Memorial Day, I had a call from the hospital. Valery, one of the nurses, sensing that I would think it was bad news, hastened to assure me that all was well; in fact the news was good. They had discontinued Lithium and were trying Loxitane instead. He was responding very well, was not nearly so tense, and much easier to handle. This was to be the beginning of a long plateau for Dave—whether it was the effect of the medication, or whether this coincided with a natural plateau, is not clear. At any rate, they were able to stabilize him with a minimum dosage of Loxitane for about a year. True, there were bad days, indifferent days, days when he was more out of touch, but overall there was no drastic degeneration. His appetite has remained good all along.

Summer was slipping by and in my own life there were changes, as I was planning to move soon into a new house, and our old home in which we had lived for thirteen years was to be rented. Dave's niece Donna was married in June, so I went down for the wedding and stayed a week with Ruth and Nolan. At the end of June, Ruth came to stay, and together we went to see Dave. It was her first experience with this ward, and she found it hard, not surprisingly. Although it was no longer possible to take him to a restaurant, he could still go out for drives and walks and still got pleasure from seeing Star whenever I brought him with me.

I was also planning to go back to England for three weeks in early September, so July was exceptionally busy, getting ready to move into the new house and for this trip to England. Everything seemed to happen at once—one of our rental houses needed painting, and this coincided with my move, so it meant much coming and going between the two houses. Worst of all were the decisions to be made when cleaning out our old house. Dave had collected endless souvenirs, photos, letters, odds and ends, much of which was junk and had to be thrown away. Nevertheless, many of these things had much sentimental value and brought back memories of happier times together. We had spent the major part of our married life in this house, so there was much nostalgia associated with it. I finally moved in on August 5, which was a Monday, and the following weekend was due for another visit to Dave. I was feeling both physically and emotionally exhausted during August, so much so that I really had no enthusiasm for my upcoming trip. Everything seemed to be an effort, and I dreaded being away from Dave for three weeks. I had very mixed feelings as to whether I should go at all and would have been thankful if something had come up to prevent it.

There are so many small details to be thought of before

leaving for a holiday—arrangements for the dogs to be taken care of, for the house to be checked periodically, mail to be stopped, decisions as to what clothes to take—the list seemed endless. For the past seven months, I had been driving a round trip of 300 miles to see him every ten days, and of course these drives were often wearing and monotonous, as well as sad. My plane would leave September 10 from Seattle, so I drove up two days before to have some time with Dave before leaving, and stayed with Harriet. When that Monday morning came, I can remember sitting on my bed at Harriet's house and breaking down again from sheer exhaustion and emotional strain.

The flight was four hours late leaving Seattle. Harriet and I had a leisurely dinner at the airport, and my spirits rose somewhat now that the responsibilities of home were left behind. Once on board, I felt better and the break from an exhausting routine was definitely needed. The three weeks passed quickly and it was a real luxury to be completely free of day-to-day chores and decision-making, and just enjoy family and friends. Meredith, the head nurse, had my sister's phone number in England in case there should be any emergency, but there was no need, for on my return, Dave was just about the same.

There had been a major change, though, for Louise, as Bill had become seriously ill with pneumonia and died the morning after I got back. She called Harriet to tell her the news while we were having breakfast. So one of my friends would not be returning to visit on that ward regularly. She would be greatly missed by staff and patients, alike, for her volunteer work on the ward had been outstanding, and her loyalty and concern for Bill and the other patients had been an example to us all.

October came, and with it a letter from Dr. Zem asking my permission for a spinal tap to be done on Dave. This would be carried out at the V.A. Hospital in Seattle sometime in November. The reason for this was to check and see if an abnormal buildup of spinal fluid in the brain was causing additional damage and loss of cells. Frankly, the idea appalled me, and I knew that Dave had always dreaded the thought of a spinal tap. However, I went at length into this with Dr. Zem, and he assured me that the risk was low. He might have some discomfort for a couple of days, but otherwise it was not a major operation. They would need him in the hospital two days beforehand, and two or three days afterwards to take some more scan pictures.

He was admitted to the neurology ward on the Saturday before Thanksgiving. Harriet had been down to stay with me, so we traveled back together and I stayed with her from Saturday till the following Wednesday. I saw Dave three times. The first time was the Sunday after his admission. I was appalled to find him sitting in a chair, unshaven, his feet bare, and only a light blanket over his pajamas. To me, it was devastating, but I am not sure how aware he was of what was going on, because he didn't seem depressed or unhappy, and greeted me with a smile and a wave as he always did. I stayed with him for about two hours and helped him with his lunch. When I asked why he had not been shaved, they told me they were very short-staffed that day, so I shaved him myself. A nurse came at my request and brought some warm socks and slippers for his feet.

The spinal tap had been scheduled for Monday morning early, and Harriet had kindly offered to go over with me to see him Monday afternoon. Although still groggy from sedation, he recognized me and we were able to go down with him to the nuclear medicine department while the scan pictures were being taken. It meant so much to be able to do this—just to share a small part of his life and experience while in the hospital. I think our presence there reassured him as he was quite responsive, smiled and tried to talk a little.

The last time I saw him on the neurology ward was the Wednesday before Thanksgiving. He had recovered really well and was able to walk up and down the ward with me. It did my heart good to see him back again to his former self; also to know that the day after Thanksgiving he would be returning to his "home base," the familiar ward at the Tacoma hospital. Dr. Zem later told me that the scan pictures had not showed any abnormal fluid buildup.

During the time he had been in Seattle, the patients on the Tacoma ward had been moved to another building, as Ward 85B was going to be remodeled. The building that would be their temporary home faced east across the lake with a magnificent view of Mt. Rainier. It was surrounded by tall firs, rhododendrons, and other colorful spring-flowering shrubs. Since the country around the hospital was mostly forest, it was quite common to see deer and also racoons in the early morning and at dusk. In fact, some of the patients fed the racoons and made pets of them. The head nurse, Meredith, told me that Dave recognized the staff on his return from Seattle—it must have been a relief to him to be back once more among faces that were familiar.

The following week was his fifty-fifth birthday, and Vinton and Maria came up for the day to celebrate with us. I bought a cake which would be shared with all those on the ward, and Harriet helped with the party. We made the most of the occasion, and I am sure this was something that meant more to us than to the men. Vint and Maria stayed to have dinner with us afterwards before driving home.

I asked Meredith one day how aware she thought Dave was and she replied, "They fade in and out like an old radio with worn-out connections." I think this is a very apt description. It's a world that we cannot enter, and most frustrating to staff and relatives alike, because communication is so limited. These men cannot express their feelings, physical pain, hunger, thirst, or other needs except by gesture and expression. That is why it is so important for the staff to be perceptive and aware of their non-verbal messages. At the same time, this makes it one of the most difficult and demanding forms of nursing. I admire those who have been able to work on this ward for two or three years—sometimes longer—and who still come back consistently. I wonder how they avoid being overcome by depression, and although they fulfill a vital role in keeping these men well maintained, the rewards are very limited as these patients are not getting any better. It takes a special kind of dedication to work on this ward for any length of time.

As Christmas approached, I had spells of depression myself and as always, this season is one of the most difficult when one is alone. The preparations seem so meaningless when there is no

161

one to share it with. I was fortunate in that Harriet invited me to spend these four days with her and her family. She also had a long-time friend, Margie, staying and the celebrations at Harriet's house were joyous and fun-filled despite our circumstances.

On Christmas Day, Margie, Harriet, and I went over to the ward and had lunch with our husbands. Dave was quite calm, I remember, and seemed fairly well in touch with things, but Les was extremely hostile and difficult, so Harriet had a sad day. We both felt so much for her and did our best to comfort her and lift her spirits. These "bad" days on the ward are devastating, as we wives know so well.

Nineteen eighty started out with another ice storm. It was the second week in January when one Tuesday afternoon, the overnight rain which had been mild was suddenly turned to sleet by a bitter east wind. By late afternoon, it was beginning to form ice on the trees and power lines. After the experience of the previous year, I took this warning seriously and built a blazing fire, knowing that most likely we were in for a major power failure. Sure enough, about 7:30 P.M., the lights flickered off and on . . . then off again for good, as ice-laden branches began crashing down. The freezing rain continued all night, and it was one of the most terrifying nights I have ever spent. I was alone in my house with the two dogs, listening to the sounds of devastation outside. Any moment I expected a branch to crash through the roof, as my house was surrounded by trees, and it was impossible to tell where the next one would fall. When some of the bigger limbs hit the ground, they shook the house to its foundations. The scene next morning was unbelievable. The driveway was completely blocked with fallen branches, and almost all the trees had sustained major damage. The power was not restored until three days later, and the telephone was off for two weeks because of a broken cable. By some miracle the roof was not badly damaged, though there were several broken tiles.

It must have been shortly after this that I decided to cut my visits to Tacoma to twice a month. The wear and tear of this journey three times a month with its accompanying emotional stress was beginning to tell on me. It was not that my loyalty to Dave was any the less—in fact, the bond had grown stronger with time—but the point had now been reached where I was sure his awareness of time was nil; that is to say, he had no concept of the passage of time between my visits.

I realized now that I would have to pick up the threads of my own life and try to do something constructive that would occupy my time and take my mind off his problem. I began to think about a part-time job which would bring a new dimension to my life, and in April took a training course with the Visiting Nurse Association to qualify as a home-health aide. I started work the end of May, doing house calls, but most of the time I have worked for one couple who need help twice weekly for three hours. Since the husband suffered a stroke, and has since been diagnosed as having Alzheimer's Disease, I have been able to give some comfort and support to his wife in how to handle this.

On my visits to Tacoma, I would usually stay with Harriet, or at a motel if I brought Star with me. Quite often, we would meet with Louise for dinner, and when on the ward with our husbands, would arrange to feed them lunch or dinner at the same table. Gradually, Dave was losing the ability to feed himself. Up till now, if I picked up the dishes and handed him a spoon, he would feed himself, but now he would often take a couple of mouthfuls, forget what he was doing and put the spoon down. One thing I am profoundly grateful for: even at this advanced stage of the disease, he was still not incontinent during the day, although he was at night. For a long time, Harriet had had to deal with this problem with Les, and often his clothes would have to be changed several times a day. It was a blessing that Dave had been spared this complication until much further along in the disease.

By now, the ward had become a part of my life, and I was no longer so appalled or repulsed by the things that I saw there. With no fears to hold me back, acceptance became much easier, and it was a challenge to try to get through to Dave on the days when he was less responsive. Often, there seemed to be an unspoken signal as to when he was receptive, and I suppose this is

163

a kind of instinct one picks up—a sort of intuition as to when is the right time to speak—when I am most likely to get an answer, a smile, a gesture that shows he is with me, and for that brief moment, has understood. His speech now was down to short phrases: "Hi, love," "Let's go," or when I asked him if he had enjoyed his meal, "Yes, I did." Interestingly, although these patients often cannot speak when asked a question, they do seem to understand a direction or request, and will obey without answering verbally.

Ruth came up again in May of 1980, and I suppose she saw a more marked deterioration in Dave than I did, as it had been almost a year since her last visit. He was going through a bad phase during that time, and when we walked him outside in the grounds he seemed very dazed and unsteady; his balance was beginning to be affected. I have a vivid remembrance of a beautiful May day, when Ruth and I were trying to get Dave to sit still long enough to admire the view across the lake, when from behind came a cheerful, familiar voice, "Hullo, you two." I looked around and saw Harriet, a courageous figure in a white skirt and navy blazer, wheeling Les in his wheelchair; he was no longer strong enough to walk any distance, so the wheelchair was a good way of getting him out for some fresh air. I don't know why this remembrance of Harriet stays with me, but I believe it was a symbol of her courage and cheerfulness which I had always admired so much.

By this time, Dave knew Louise and Harriet really well, since they were more often on the ward than I was. He would greet both of them affectionately, and on one occasion, asked Louise if she would go to Hawaii with him!

May 25, 1980 was a Sunday, and I decided to leave the house early, so as to get up to the hospital by lunch time. I had not listened to the news that morning, and as I left the sky was gray and overcast. Soon afterwards, it started to rain, but this rain was heavy, thick, and stuck to the windshield like snow-flakes. The farther north I went, the worse it became. Then the realization dawned that I was driving through the results of a volcanic eruption. The road conditions grew steadily worse and my tires were now grinding through a slimy, brown glue, skidding from time to time, and the sky was so dark it could have been midnight. I pulled in thankfully at the small town of Kelso, and stopped at a gas station to wash off the car. Other drivers were passing through from the north, and I asked how it was—the answer was always the same—it's really bad. Kelso was without lights or heat. Should I turn and drive the forty-odd miles back again, or should I go on? I felt that, having got this far, it would be no worse going on than going back; either way it was a risk. The rest of that journey was a nightmare. I was trembling and praying for protection during the next sixty miles or so. I saw many cars pull off the road and give up, and thought that at any moment this would be my fate too. By some miracle, the car kept going, even though the windshield washers had long since given up and the wipers were so clogged they could barely clear enough space to see through. Once I had to stop in the middle of the freeway (I couldn't see enough to pull off to the side of the road) and wipe the windows off with a towel. Farther on, the rain had stopped, but now there was dry swirling ash, as fine as face powder, seeping into everything. It was blowing like a dust storm across the highway, and the slightest movement kicked it up into clouds. I drove as fast as I dared. *Surely, there will be an end to this before too long.* As I looked out of the windows, I was horrified to see that the trees were laden down with a coating of heavy, gray ash; also the animals out grazing in the fields were covered, and so of course, was the grass they were eating. About twenty-five miles south of the hospital, the ash fall gradually lessened and the sun broke through, so the last stage of my journey was easy.

How I made it through I will never know. The car was completely covered with ash—it had filtered into the engine also, and I had to take it in and get the motor steam-cleaned the next day. I stayed up an extra day with Harriet that time, as conditions were still bad on the roads. However, on my arrival at the hospital I got a very special reward. Dave was sitting at the table eating his lunch when I walked in. His face lit up, he waved and shouted "Hullo," and motioned me to come and sit down with him. Such are the rewards in a situation like this; my drive through

165

the volcanic ash had been more than worthwhile.

The second week in June, Harriet and I shared a table for lunch with Les and Dave, as usual. As I remember, it was one of the good days for us both, since our husbands were quite alert, and I think we even had a few laughs. That was to be the last time we would be together for a meal on the ward. The Sunday following, June 15, Les died. Earlier that spring, he had pneumonia which had weakened him considerably, and later he had problems swallowing. It was difficult to get him to eat as the muscles which controlled swallowing were now affected. He was taken in his sleep one night, and this had been an answer to Harriet's prayers. Up to the end, he had still been able to walk around on the ward, so was spared the lengthy, slow deterioration which sometimes happens.

Vinton came up to the funeral with me as Dave's representative. He and I and Louise drove to the church together that sunny June afternoon to pay our last respects to Les, together with Harriet and her family. Needless to say, it was an emotional time, but above all there has to be thankfulness for the way he left this world—that is what we would wish for all those we love.

Now I made my visits to the ward without the support of Harriet and Louise. It was not easy, but I still felt a protective veil surrounding my feelings, so I was able to cope, and my visits to him would always have priority. I had the feeling that he would know me right up to the end.

In September, the patients were due to be moved back to Ward 85B, which was now finished and repainted. The date was set for September 17, so I went up the day before to be there in time to help on moving day. When I arrived at the ward, things were chaotic, because almost all of the furniture except for bare necessities had been moved already; the patients were upset because of all the confusion, and Dave was worse than I had seen him for a long time. He wandered around in a daze, not giving any sign of recognition, looking gaunt and haggard; that day he could not speak, except to make a grunting noise in the back of his throat. I was so overcome that I had to leave the ward, and go down to sit by the lake for a while. The surroundings were so

166

peaceful compared to the turmoil I had just left and the sorrow in my own heart. Tears welled up within me and overflowed. My defenses, which I once thought were so strong, had broken down. There was no solution for the moment but to weep it all out of my system; when the tears had expressed what could not be said in words, then I would be healed again and ready once more to face my tragedy.

That evening, I talked to Louise, who was also going over to help with the move. We planned to meet at the hospital, and when we arrived, the men had already been assembled in a downstairs room to wait until final preparations on the remodeled ward were complete. This day was altogether different; because the room is quiet without the turmoil of moving, they are quiet too. Dave greeted me and was quite responsive. It was such a help having Louise and Mim, one of the other wives, there for mutual support. Shortly after lunch we were told that the new ward was now ready, so we all went up, patients, staff, and wives, to resume life once more in new surroundings. Those patients who could still walk—Dave and four or five of the others—immediately began to wander up and down, taking stock of their new home. Louise and Mim and I helped unpacking clothes and putting them away, which took about two hours. It was good to have something to do that made us feel useful. Having helped feed dinner to the patients, we joined Harriet and Charlotte for dinner. These evenings with the other wives were always a source of comfort to me—it was a time to relax and if possible, forget the trauma of the ward. To share some jokes, or talk about things that had no connection with the tragedies of our lives.

The day room in the remodeled ward is decorated in sunny colors of orange and yellow. There is a green plant hanging in each window and hanging plants also adorn the nurses' station, which is blue and white. Most of the patients' rooms are painted white with different colored curtains in each room. Dave now shares a four-bed room with three other patients at about the same stage.

As of September, 1980, his long plateau without much change came to an end, and he started once more to deteriorate. He

167

would no longer walk straight up and down the length of the ward, as previously, but paced in small circles, usually leaning to the right. When I tried to walk him outside, he did the same thing and didn't really seem comfortable or to get enjoyment from being out. As the disease worsens, familiar surroundings become ever more important. He had started to lose weight too; when he first came on the ward in January 1979 he weighed 162 pounds. As of January 1981, he was down to 139. Loxitane, which had stabilized him so well for the past year or so, no longer seemed to be effective, so he was switched to a minimum dose of Haldol instead. The dose would be adjusted according to his mood of the day—if he was reasonably calm, then it might be reduced, if he was tense and agitated, it would be increased. Always, though, the staff tried to strike a balance, to find the level at which the drug would have beneficial effects without extreme drowsiness. I was impressed by the way they had been able to adjust constantly to Dave's changes by working to find just the right dosage to keep him comfortable, but not out of touch.

Twice since the move back to the remodeled ward, I took him out for a drive. It was difficult getting him in and out of the car, as he didn't seem to understand what we were trying to do; also his legs and whole body were very stiff now, and he had problems bending down and swinging his legs over to the front of the seat. Once in the car, however, he still seemed to enjoy the motion and was fairly relaxed. We stopped at Louise's apartment for a few minutes and she came out to see him. He tried to get out, and we had considerable difficulty getting him back in again. I noticed as we drove along how frail he looked, and how stooped his posture had become.

We had a good Thanksgiving together. I arrived in time for lunch and we went into the visitors' room with our trays. Dave was quite alert and responded well; he did his best to have conversation with me, and what he couldn't say in words was conveyed by his expression and gestures. As we got up to leave after lunch, he banged into a chair and toppled over on to the floor. Fortunately I was holding him by both hands and was able to pull him up without too much trouble. So even at this late date, there were still rewards, still communication, but of a totally different kind.

How long will this journey go on? As those who have experienced Alzheimer's Disease will know, there is no logical sequence to the ups and downs, and the disease does not progress in a way that can be predicted with any accuracy. I pray that when the final stage does come for Dave, it will not mean a long period of total helplessness, but if this should be the case, then I have to learn to adjust in the same way that I have to all the other changes.

In early January, all medication was discontinued for about a week to see what the effects would be. When I came up to visit at that time, he looked very thin and when sitting in his chair would have convulsive movements. I asked Meredith about this, and she said it was the result of having no medication at all; they would wait until all traces of the drug were out of his system before trying something new. Next he was on a minimum dosage of Narvane and Cogentin. Surprisingly, he still ate well and seemed to enjoy his food; however, he did have swallowing problems from time to time.

He still knows me—runs to greet me when I appear on the ward. In spite of the ravages of this dreadful disease, there is a noticeable dignity about him which to me is an answer to prayer. Dear God, don't let him go through the gruesome final stages, but take him peacefully in his asleep. May his first night's welcome home in heaven be very special.

9. Hope and Encouragement

So far, this has been a book dealing with tragedy, stark tragedy in the life of someone who had to face a terminal disease much too early. I shall probably never know in this life why he had to face this—why it was allowed to cross our path. But face it we had to; there was no possible escape.

In this chapter I want to explore the ways in which I found hope; I cannot of course speak for Dave because so much of the time he was not in touch with my kind of reality. Hope is hard to define, but it is also difficult to kill. It seems to exist in spite of ourselves in the darkest of situations. It appears unexpectedly as a promise that all is not lost—things are not as they seem on the surface. There is a deeper meaning.

This reassurance grew stronger the further we went into the crisis. To begin with, there is a feeling that this has a purpose. It is doing things in my life and perhaps in the lives of others which would not have happened otherwise. There is a special closeness between family and friends which far surpasses our usual routine exchanges. It deepens and enlarges our relationships. Of course this happening is something we would never choose for ourselves, but through it new heights are reached, new courage is found, endurance and stamina are built up.

We learn to reach out and live on a different level than before. It confirms to me that our lives are watched over by our Creator. Each moment is of importance. We are not asked to look ahead, but only to live each day as it comes. Encouragement is the realization that we are not forsaken—there will always be provision for our needs, even in the darkest times. True, there will be times when the future is obscured and we cannot see one inch of the way ahead. But in living through such times, there are always consolations to be found. A good friend drops in for a visit. There is music to listen to, animals to enjoy, an unexpected reason to laugh. The seasons pass as they always have; the sun still rises each morning, birds sing, and the smell of a summer rose in full bloom drenches the air.

Perhaps for me one of the greatest consolations was that Dave showed more love and tenderness toward me as his condition grew worse. He was open and vulnerable now in a way that he never had been before. Although it seemed ironic that this should happen now, at a time when he was losing his other faculties, I realized I had to accept it and be grateful.

Friends were another source of great comfort and support. I can honestly say that at no time was I ever without someone to turn to in time of need. It takes a while to be able to see beyond the blackness to signs of hope like these, but they are there and they are real.

When we first had the diagnosis, it was almost impossible to find hope anywhere—the enormity and horror of it devastated life for the time being. Initially, I felt sure he would be healed, that God would not allow this to happen. This I now realize came as a blessing to take away the pangs of the first, terrible shock. Partly, it was not facing up to reality—a reality I wasn't ready for yet.

We tried to put off or deny reality during our trip to England in the fall of 1976. It was a last attempt to prove to ourselves that it could be done. True, there were many anxious moments and difficulties, awkward, embarrassing times for us both when we realized he was just not capable of adapting and taking part in life over there. It showed his limitations all too clearly, and yet there were happy moments too. Hope and encouragement were found in the loyalty of friends and family who accepted us with all the complications and never failed to show their love and concern.

171

As things gradually grew worse, I was still not facing reality. It was too cruel, too unbelievable to think that at the age of fifty-one he was deteriorating so rapidly. My next phase of hope came in actively searching for a solution. Maybe we were meant to find an answer outside traditional medicine, and his healing would be our reward. When he responded so well to the acupuncture treatments, our hearts were lifted once more. It seemed that the miracle we had prayed for might be in sight, within our grasp, against all the odds, all the predictions against such a cure.

As has been indicated earlier in this book, acupuncture provided a remission which was real and for the time being prospects were that the improvement might be maintained. I now have to ask myself the question: Why were we given this hope, this reprieve, only to have it fade again and have to face the original diagnosis? What was being done during that time of remission to strengthen us for what we had to face next?

I see in the remission a hope that one day there will be a way to arrest, possibly even to reverse the disease. Who knows how long it will be? Ten years, fifteen, twenty years? But I am convinced that there will be an answer. It will not come soon enough to help us, but perhaps the information that comes from Dave's brain, or the brain of someone else on the research ward, will provide the clue that is vital.

I have to be thankful for the fact that Dave was given those three months in which he was able to enjoy life and return to a point where he was well enough to go for a job interview, to drive himself without my help, to have some measure of independence and fulfillment. I have to believe that even in his helpless, defenseless state—a life to all appearances without meaning—that there is a reason. Why is he allowed to live on if there is no purpose? What is there that we cannot see or understand which still keeps him alive when to all intents and purposes he leads an empty existence? I cannot believe that life is ever wasted, but there are still possibilities for growth in even (outwardly) the most hopeless situations.

I feel that prayers have been answered in that even though severely handicapped as he is now, there is still a kind of poise about him, a peace and serenity. He often smiles or waves to those he sees nearby, and even though his speech is almost gone, he occasionally gets out a sentence that is not garbled. The fact that he still remembers me makes the whole difference to my visits. It is an assurance that the bond between us is still there, and I think it always will be, right up to the end.

Although we are so far apart in distance, I know now that this is the right place for him to be. It is the best possible care he could have under such circumstances. I look back two years and remember how much I dreaded this move, my fear of the upheaval it would bring once more into our lives. And yet . . . it has proved to be the most constructive thing that could have happened. Through it, I have learned to accept this ward and to be thankful for what is being done there. I have also gained two outstanding friends whose loyalty and support have been invaluable.

If I cannot get through to him in words, then there is still touch, and when I tell him that I love him, there is often a response: "I know you do." How much do my visits mean to him? One of the nurses told me that they really sustained him, and that he did his very best to act normally while I was there. When talking to Harriet on the phone, I am encouraged when she has been over to see her husband and tells me that Dave greeted her and that he looked clean and neat, freshly shaved with clean clothes. Perhaps she will tell me what he was wearing today. What a comfort. From this distance any small items of news such as this make my day and give me renewed strength. Some of the other patients on the ward recognize me and those who are able say hullo and often we have some conversation.

I realize that gradually, almost imperceptibly, my dread of hospital visiting has been replaced by acceptance and coming to know those who live and work there as friends, as part of my life. The day-to-day happenings on the ward are of real interest; it gives me pleasure to listen to an account of what a patient has said or done; to chat with a nurse and perhaps listen to some of her frustrations and feelings about this difficult and demanding job. The rewards are few but they are there in the form of nursing a patient through a serious illness to the point where he can once again respond within his limits. Even those who are really far gone will often have days when they are quite alert and can get out a word or a smile.

There is a bond between us—a bond of interest and caring, of learning a totally new kind of communication with those who can no longer speak or express their own needs. We learn to watch their expressions which usually signal the mood of the moment. How to touch and guide them to the dinner table. How to make them sit down, how to change their clothes or take them to the bathroom. Touch is so very important as often it is the only communication left.

One of the aides, Debbie, told me that one night she had a real struggle getting Dave undressed and ready for bed. He resisted her all the way, was uncooperative and abusive. Finally, when she got him into bed and was about to leave the room, he looked up at her and said, "Thank you for taking care of me."

Ruth and I were helping Dave with his lunch on the ward one day, when suddenly he said, "I saw Susan last night." Susan was his niece who was in California at that time, so we just wrote it off as a passing thought that had crossed his mind. When we got back to my house, Ruth telephoned Susan and told her what Dave had said. She said, "It's true, I saw him in a dream last night; he was sitting in a chair and I went over and hugged him."

When I meet one of the other wives on the ward, there is an immediate unspoken understanding between us. We have been brought together here for some unknown reason. Most likely our paths would never have crossed if it hadn't been for Ward 85B.

The most valuable lifesaver of all is laughter. I am so grateful to Louise and Harriet for teaching me, by their example, to see the funny side of things. We could laugh often about some of the things our husbands said or did—not laughing at them, but seeing humor which helped to make us more relaxed, to bring a situation into perspective. Sometimes we were even able to laugh at ourselves. The things we thought were so important or so painful would be dissolved completely for the moment. How vital a sense of humor is. When we look back on our times together during that devastating period of our lives, what will stand out? What will last? It will be different for each of us, but for me I am sure it will be the times when laughter was shared unexpectedly during a day when I felt nothing but grief.

We have so much to learn from life. Slowly and painfully, I have learned not to run away from the darkness it brings; this experience has helped me to overcome a fear of the unknown which I have had for years, long before I was married to Dave. I am confident that when this phase of my life is over, this nameless dread will be gone forever. I too, will have been healed, though in a way I would never have chosen myself.

As time went on, I learned to enjoy my outings with him, limited though they were. I have not been able to take him to a restaurant for two years now, but up until the spring of 1980, he could still go out for a drive. Occasionally, I can take him out for a walk when the weather is good, but this is not easy now as he seldom walks straight, leans heavily to the right and keeps changing direction. Our little dog, Star, gave him great pleasure for a long time and added spice to our walks. Now he is seldom able to focus long enough to realize that Star is there.

One day in November 1979, Louise kindly invited us over to her apartment for lunch. We decided we would have to play it by ear, and if he was very restless, I would obviously have to take him back. It worked out beautifully. He responded warmly to Louise, seemed to recognize her, and relaxed at once in her armchair. He was able to eat lunch at the table with us without any help and really enjoyed his meal. Afterwards he sat down again in the armchair and went to sleep for a while. He understood what Louise was saying most of the time and responded appropriately. These kinds of things are a triumph when they work out well, and on such triumphs my life is built now. They are rewards along the way that are very special.

My heart is lifted when he runs to greet me on the ward with a big hug—sometimes he will reach up and touch my face for a moment; he seems to be trying to imprint it on his memory. On days when he has been off in his own world for a long time and I despair of getting any response, he will suddenly look up and say "Hullo, love." Words do not come easily now and often

175

it is an effort for him to talk. When this happens, I just hold his hand and tell him I love him.

I am confident that there will be rewards right up to the end if I can remain open and perceptive enough to recognize them. In continuing to visit on a regular basis (twice a month) I am still learning that communication without words can be real and have a lot of meaning. In a way it's like breaking through a barrier that I would have once thought impossible. I get pleasure from feeding him, helping to change his clothes, even taking him to the bathroom. It's enough just to be there and know that I am sharing in these small everyday things.

I think ahead to the time when he will go on to the next world, when he will be transformed into a new being, all suffering wiped away, tears and tragedy a thing of the past. One day, when spending a weekend with friends in Idaho, we took a drive from Boise up to Sun Valley. It was in late October, and there had been some snow the night before. Sunshine and shadow chased each other in ever-varying shades of gold and blue across the immense landscape. In the far distance, the sky shaded almost to black where showers still lingered, and the distant mountains were sharply etched against the horizon. The air was crystal clear and the view uninterrupted by any sign of human life. Just the peace and tranquility of mile after mile of open rangeland stretching away as far as the eye could see in every direction.

On our way back that evening, the scene was even more impressive. As twilight came on, there was an air of mystery, as the brilliant colors of midday faded and softened to a rosy hue and then a purplish brown on the mountains. The sun was setting in a bank of black clouds away to the west, spreading a reddish glow which gradually faded to pink, then pale gold and finally eggshell blue before darkness fell. The colors shrouding the fields were soft, grayish green, dusky, smoke-colored in the distance with always that purple shadow on the distant hills. Twilight seemed to linger long in that high country with a beauty that was outstanding. All around was space, space, and more space of an almost indescribable splendor, unmarred by civilization, complete and whole and satisfying in itself.

As we drove along in silence, it came to me that perhaps heaven will be something like this scene—all the beauty, the loveliness we have ever experienced here on earth will be found in heaven, though in a different dimension and on an infinitely grander scale. I like to think that times such as these when we enjoy something so moving, so great that it defies description, are sent to give us a glimpse of what is to come. I am sure the Almighty constantly gives us glimpses, visions like this if we are aware enough to understand their message.

And so, I long for the time when Dave will one day experience this place of unbelievable beauty, peace and harmony. Does he too have his own visions of this world to come? The fact that this may be so is one of my greatest sources of hope now. It is not something that can be proved scientifically, but I have within me a deep inner assurance that what he suffers now will be turned into glory, triumph, and victory in a way that can only be felt, not explained.

One day, probably not in this life, but in the next, I will see the whole picture of our lives, understand the reasons why we had to go through this—I will be able to see Dave's life in perspective, and there will be answers to the now-unanswered questions. There will be enlightenment and wholeness, yet we will see the true value of what we lived through here on earth and will know that none of it was wasted.

> For we know in part and we prophesy in part
> But when that which is perfect is come
> Then that which is in part shall be done away
>
> For now we see through a glass darkly
> But then face to face. Now I know in part,
> But then shall I know even as also I am known.

Epilogue

It is Palm Sunday, 1982. A crystal-clear spring day, with bright sunshine flooding through the windows as I visit the ward where now nine of the nineteen patients are in wheelchairs because they can no longer walk. Recently, Dave joined this group. Progressively, for about the last month or so, his walking had been getting worse until it was no longer safe to let him walk alone. As I sit beside his chair, I am struggling to accept this change, the change I have dreaded the most. The ward is very quiet this morning, as though the promise of spring has spread an aura of peace within these walls, where the struggle for life goes on unceasingly twenty-four hours a day.

It is too much effort for me even to talk to the staff or make any attempt to hide my grief; it surrounds me like a pall as I try to grasp the reality that this change in him is final and our days of walking up and down the ward together are now a thing of the past. There is something so very irrevocable about this downturn; it's almost like going back to the time when we first had the diagnosis and learning to relive acceptance all over again.

He is almost totally helpless, rigid, and a dead weight who has to be lifted up in his chair as he can no longer support himself or adjust to any change of position alone. However, he seems quite cheerful—smiles and sometimes laughs and still recognizes me. His eyes are bright and full of expression and his smile spontaneous. There is something in the smile of a severely handicapped person that turns the heart upside down. Perhaps because it is such an expression of triumph over all that can afflict the body. By what miracle is he still able to have a sense of humor now with so little of his mind left intact?

For a long time, I have prayed that he not be allowed to go through the final stages of this disease, plagued with bedsores, unable to swallow, and enduring other complications characteristic of this advanced stage. An awful fear grips me that perhaps, after all, he will have to go the full course, but I dare not dwell on this as it would destroy me. A new stage of growth has arrived for me too—I have to learn not to dwell on his condition and what lies ahead or how long it will be. I sense that once again I will not be allowed to suffer the full force of this disaster. Plumbing the depths is not for me because those depths lie beyond what I, as a human being, can bear. The bond between us is still strong and I know that I must continue to see him even though my times at the hospital will be shorter now as there is so little I can do. If I can steel myself to fly into the teeth of this tragedy, I will not be overcome and the sting of grief will lose its power.

My love for him is just as strong as it ever was, in a way I could never have imagined. But it must not be a possessive love that would seek to hold him back when the time has come for him to move out of this life; it must be a love that looks on my personal loss as something to be experienced gladly because for him it will be a release from a body that can no longer function, and the beginning of real life free from the sorrows of this world forever.

Five months have passed and September is here—eighteen years ago this month we were married, little knowing where our journey through life would take us. It is a cloudy, damp day with more than a hint of fall in the air as I visit the ward on a Saturday afternoon. For several weeks now he has been off all medication and his alertness and responsiveness have definitely improved. Although he can no longer talk, he often seems to understand what I tell him or ask him, and will sometimes nod and smile when I mention someone he was once close to, such

179

as his parents or a good friend. Today I have brought with me some tapes of choral music, the Tabernacle choir, some Beethoven, Pavarotti singing Christmas carols. I know by his expression that they give him pleasure. There is a peace, a tranquility about him, and his eyes mirror the transcendent joy of this music.

The staff tells me that some days he is able to walk quite well (supported on either side, of course), so it appears that he may be on another plateau for a while. I notice too that his swallowing at mealtimes has improved, although all his food is pureed now. For me, this pattern of visiting every two weeks has become a way of life now; it's hard to remember a time when it wasn't this way. I have been able to accept what I expect to be the final change, and not think about it. I just concentrate on the times when his eyes light up and show me that we are still communicating.

In a recent edition of the A.D.R.D.A.* newsletter, Dr. Benson Schaeffer, a Portland psychologist, wrote:

Many readers have asked the question: How much is the person with Alzheimer's disease aware of his/her incapacities? There is no easy answer but there are at least two ways of approaching the question. (1) We can try to understand the nature of the memory losses which are usually present, and (2) we can learn to respect the wholeness of the person's psychological world.

Regarding memory losses, the important point to be kept in mind is that such losses inevitably interfere with awareness. The person who does not remember events, people, places, things, and facts does not remember that he/she does not remember. Partial memories may remain, and along with them a partial awareness of incapacities, but complete awareness is usually not possible. This may be a good thing.

Regarding the private psychological world of the person with Alzheimer's disease, we can only make educated

---

*Ahzheimer's Disease and Related Disorders Association.

guesses. It is my impression, however, that their world can have a considerable unity, a comfortable wholeness and integration—that it need not be a black world. The unity I envision is based more on a positive, integrated emotional tone than on understanding through language. In our attempts at empathy we often assume that our own negative feelings accurately mirror the problem experienced by the person with Alzheimer's disease. This is very likely an incorrect assumption. Trying to bring your view of things to the person with Alzheimer's disease may not be possible and it may not be appreciated.

This has been of great comfort to me as it confirms what I have felt myself, namely that Dave's world may not necessarily be a sad one. For him, being so far removed from the struggles of everyday life just may have been a blessing. I venture even further to suggest that, although obviously there are "bad" days, "uncomfortable" days, as there are for any of us, he may now be more content in his own little world than he has ever been before. As I mentioned earlier, it often seemed that he was overwhelmed by the blows and failures of his life and was unable to rise above them. Could this stage then, be a time of peace and preparation where he is able to relax and enjoy himself to some extent, free from all stress, from the demands of trying to make a success of life in worldly terms?

He walks a path I cannot see
Shrouded deep in its own mystery
For reasons I shall never know
His mind was taken away and so,
We went down into life's dark days
Not seeing an inch of the way ahead
Not knowing whence would come the strength,
To help us live through these tortuous ways.
A way not of our choosing, but a mightier hand
Had traced the way we could not understand.
And now, though time grows short

And what we have to bear seems harder yet
Remember that the One who holds each moment of our lives
Does not forget our suffering, our agony
And as at Calvary the victory was his alone,
So this last enemy will be overthrown
In our lives too.

"For the last enemy that shall be destroyed is death."